AF687149

Physical Education, Exercise Science and Sport

Physical Education, Exercise Science and Sport

Liam Owens

Larsen & Keller
www.larsen-keller.com

Physical Education, Exercise Science and Sport
Liam Owens
ISBN: 978-1-64172-698-6 (Hardback)

© 2022 Larsen & Keller

Larsen & Keller
Published by Larsen and Keller Education,
5 Penn Plaza,
19th Floor,
New York, NY 10001, USA

Cataloging-in-Publication Data

Physical education, exercise science and sport / Liam Owens.
p. cm.
Includes bibliographical references and index.
ISBN 978-1-64172-698-6
1. Physical education and training. 2. Exercise. 3. Sports. I. Owens, Liam.
GV341 .P49 2022
613.7--dc23

This book contains information obtained from authentic and highly regarded sources. All chapters are published with permission under the Creative Commons Attribution Share Alike License or equivalent. A wide variety of references are listed. Permissions and sources are indicated; for detailed attributions, please refer to the permissions page. Reasonable efforts have been made to publish reliable data and information, but the authors, editors and publisher cannot assume any responsibility for the validity of all materials or the consequences of their use.

Trademark Notice: All trademarks used herein are the property of their respective owners. The use of any trademark in this text does not vest in the author or publisher any trademark ownership rights in such trademarks, nor does the use of such trademarks imply any affiliation with or endorsement of this book by such owners.

For more information regarding Larsen and Keller Education and its products, please visit the publisher's website www.larsen-keller.com

Table of Contents

Preface

The study of the working of a healthy human body during exercise is known as sports and exercise science. It also studies the impact of sport and physical activity on improving health, and performance from cellular to whole body perspectives. This field draws from several other disciplines such as anatomy, exercise physiology, sport psychology, biochemistry, biomechanics and biokinetics. A major application of sport and exercise science is designing, monitoring and evaluating training programs for athletes and coaches to enable them to reach their maximum potential. This book attempts to understand the multiple branches that fall under the discipline of sport and exercise science and how such concepts have practical applications. The topics included in this book on sports and exercise science, are of utmost significance and bound to provide incredible insights to readers. Those in search of information to further their knowledge will be greatly assisted by this book.

A detailed account of the significant topics covered in this book is provided below:

Chapter 1- The branch of science that studies the effects of sports and exercise on the human body is referred to as sports and exercise science. It uses the concepts of Human anatomy, human physiological systems, skeletal muscle physiology, etc. Topics elaborated in this chapter will briefly introduce about sports and exercise science.

Chapter 2- The physiology of physical science is termed as exercise physiology. Biological equilibrium of energy in the human body is called energy balance. The study of immune system is defined as immunology. The study of body movements in all organisms is defined as kinesiology. This chapter closely examines exercise physiology, immunology and kinesiology to provide an extensive understanding of the subject.

Chapter 3- Use of physics in sports is termed as physics of sports. It is a vast subject that branches out into sports biomechanics, kinematics of human motion, linear kinetics in sports, angular kinematics, fluid mechanics, sport aerodynamics, impulse and momentum, etc., which have been thoroughly discussed in this chapter.

Chapter 4- Nutrition is important for athletes to maintain the daily intake of essential nutrients. Sports nutrition is a field that aims to understand the need and impact of proper nutrition in athletes. This chapter delves into diverse aspects of nutrition with respect to sport and exercise such as supplements, multivitamins and various other energy sources.

Chapter 5- An interdisciplinary science that integrates the concepts of physiology, kinesiology, biomechanics and psychology is referred to as sports psychology.

Performance anxiety, aggression in sport, psychological susceptibility to injury, body image and self-esteem are sub-fields of this science. This chapter discusses in detail these theories related to sports psychology.

It gives me an immense pleasure to thank our entire team for their efforts. Finally in the end, I would like to thank my family and colleagues who have been a great source of inspiration and support.

Liam Owens

1

Introduction to Sport and Exercise Science

The branch of science that studies the effects of sports and exercise on the human body is referred to as sports and exercise science. It uses the concepts of Human anatomy, human physiological systems, skeletal muscle physiology, etc. Topics elaborated in this chapter will briefly introduce about sports and exercise science.

Sport and Exercise Science

Sport and exercise science is the application of scientific principles to sport and exercise, achieved through one of the following three branches of science, or through interdisciplinary approaches:

Biomechanics - An examination of the causes and consequences of human movement and the interaction of the body with apparatus or equipment through the application of mechanical principles.

Physiology - The branch of the biological sciences that is concerned with the way that the body responds to exercise and training.

Psychology - The branch of sport and exercise science that seeks to provide answers to questions about human behaviour in sport and exercise settings.

Interdisciplinary - Involves seeking to contribute to the body of knowledge or solve a real-world problem using two or more disciplines in an integrated fashion from the outset.

The science of sport and exercise attempts to answer questions such as:

- What happens to the body during physical activity?
- How and why do injuries occur?
- How does the body and mind react in extreme environments?
- What can physical activity support the prevention and treatment of chronic diseases?
- How can athletes improve their performance?

With the issue of participation in physical activity high on the political agenda and high performance sport embracing science more than ever before, the scope and demand for applying sport and exercise science in a variety of contexts is growing.

Application of Sport and Exercise Science

Sport and exercise science can be applied within a broad range of contexts. The most basic distinction that can be drawn is between its use in a 'sport science' context versus its use in an 'exercise science' context.

Sport science tends to refer to the application of sport and exercise science principles within high performance sport, where the application of science is concerned with maximising the performance of an athlete or team.

Exercise science refers to the application of sport and exercise science principles within health and fitness, where the application of science is primarily concerned with the improvement of physical and mental health through exercise. This covers both the role that exercise can play in preventing poor health and chronic diseases, such as coronary heart disease and diabetes, and the role of exercise in treating a variety of physiological and psychological disorders.

Interdisciplinary Sport and Exercise Science

Interdisciplinary sport and exercise scientists attempt to align theoretical principles with practical delivery, utilising more than one core sub-discipline of sport and exercise science (biomechanics, physiology, psychology) in an integrated and co-ordinated manner, in an attempt to solve real problems for individuals and groups within the sport and exercise environments.

This problem-based approach is based upon a realisation that:

- Performance is based upon a set of functionally inter-linking variables.
- Knowledge of how different variables inter-link is imperative and under-researched (and often in practice relies upon the role of experiential knowledge).

The skills required for this approach include:

- Bridge building - The coming together of specialist knowledge from different disciplines.
- Restructuring - Methodologies, theories and practices from one discipline are borrowed and transposed into another discipline to restructure the approach to a problem.
- Integration - The application and combination of different disciplines.

Human Anatomy

Human body is the physical substance of the human organism, composed of living cells and extracellular materials and organized into tissues, organs, and systems.

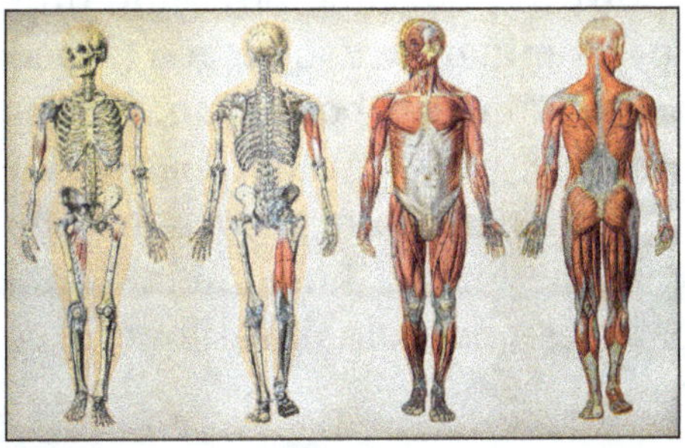

Human body; human anatomy Vintage anatomy charts of the human body showing the skeletal and muscle systems.

Humans are, of course, animals—more particularly, members of the order Primates in the subphylum Vertebrata of the phylum Chordata. Like all chordates, the human animal has a bilaterally symmetrical body that is characterized at some point during its development by a dorsal supporting rod (the notochord), gill slits in the region of the pharynx, and a hollow dorsal nerve cord. Of these features, the first two are present only during the embryonic stage in the human; the notochord is replaced by the vertebral column, and the pharyngeal gill slits are lost completely. The dorsal nerve cord is the spinal cord in humans; it remains throughout life.

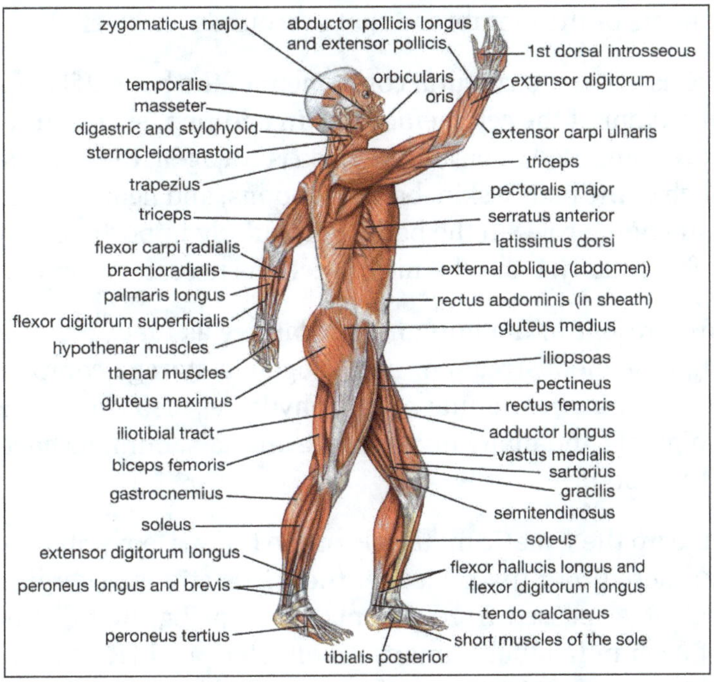

Human muscular system: Lateral view Lateral view of the human muscular system.

Characteristic of the vertebrate form, the human body has an internal skeleton that includes a backbone of vertebrae. Typical of mammalian structure, the human body shows such characteristics as hair, mammary glands, and highly developed sense organs.

Beyond these similarities, however, lie some profound differences. Among the mammals, only humans have a predominantly two-legged (bipedal) posture, a fact that has greatly modified the general mammalian body plan. (Even the kangaroo, which hops on two legs when moving rapidly, walks on four legs and uses its tail as a "third leg" when standing.) Moreover, the human brain, particularly the neocortex, is far and away the most highly developed in the animal kingdom. As intelligent as are many other mammals—such as chimpanzees and dolphins—none have achieved the intellectual status of the human species.

Chemical Composition of the Body

Chemically, the human body consists mainly of water and of organic compounds—i.e., lipids, proteins, carbohydrates, and nucleic acids. Water is found in the extracellular fluids of the body (the blood plasma, the lymph, and the interstitial fluid) and within the cells themselves. It serves as a solvent without which the chemistry of life could not take place. The human body is about 60 percent water by weight.

Lipids—chiefly fats, phospholipids, and steroids—are major structural components of the human body. Fats provide an energy reserve for the body, and fat pads also serve as insulation and shock absorbers. Phospholipids and the steroid compound cholesterol are major components of the membrane that surrounds each cell.

Proteins also serve as a major structural component of the body. Like lipids, proteins are an important constituent of the cell membrane. In addition, such extracellular materials as hair and nails are composed of protein. So also is collagen, the fibrous, elastic material that makes up much of the body's skin, bones, tendons, and ligaments. Proteins also perform numerous functional roles in the body. Particularly important are cellular proteins called enzymes, which catalyze the chemical reactions necessary for life.

Carbohydrates are present in the human body largely as fuels, either as simple sugars circulating through the bloodstream or as glycogen, a storage compound found in the liver and the muscles. Small amounts of carbohydrates also occur in cell membranes, but, in contrast to plants and many invertebrate animals, humans have little structural carbohydrate in their bodies.

Nucleic acids make up the genetic materials of the body. Deoxyribonucleic acid (DNA) carries the body's hereditary master code, the instructions according to which each cell operates. It is DNA, passed from parents to offspring, that dictates the inherited characteristics of each individual human. Ribonucleic acid (RNA), of which there are several types, helps carry out the instructions encoded in the DNA.

Along with water and organic compounds, the body's constituents include various inorganic minerals. Chief among these are calcium, phosphorus, sodium, magnesium, and iron. Calcium and phosphorus, combined as calcium-phosphate crystals, form a large part of the body's bones. Calcium is also present as ions in the blood and interstitial fluid, as is sodium. Ions of phosphorus, potassium, and magnesium, on the other hand, are abundant within the intercellular fluid. All of these ions play vital roles in the body's metabolic processes. Iron is present mainly as part of hemoglobin, the oxygen-carrying pigment of the red blood cells. Other mineral constituents of the body, found in minute but necessary concentrations, include cobalt, copper, iodine, manganese, and zinc.

Organization of the Body

The cell is the basic living unit of the human body—indeed, of all organisms. The human body consists of trillions of cells, each capable of growth, metabolism, response to stimuli, and, with some exceptions, reproduction. Although there are some 200 different types of cells in the body, these can be grouped into four basic classes. These four basic cell types, together with their extracellular materials, form the fundamental tissues of the human body: (1) epithelial tissues, which cover the body's surface and line the internal organs, body cavities, and passageways; (2) muscle tissues, which are capable of contraction and form the body's musculature; (3) nerve tissues, which conduct electrical impulses and make up the nervous system; and (4) connective tissues, which are composed of widely spaced cells and large amounts of intercellular matrix and which bind together various body structures. (Bone and blood are considered specialized connective tissues, in which the intercellular matrix is, respectively, hard and liquid).

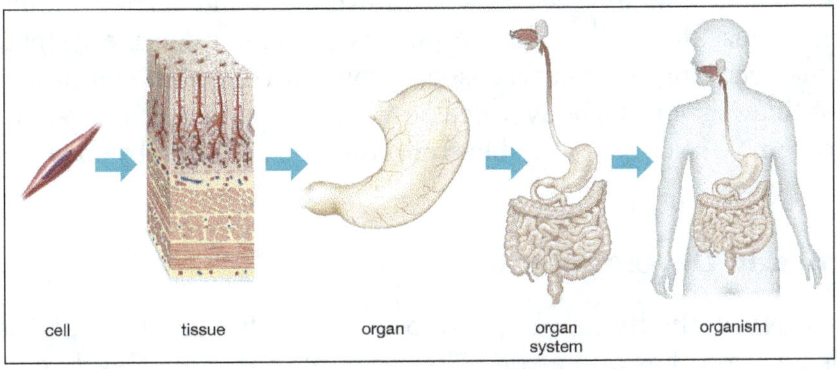

Multicelluar organism: Organization.

The diagram shows five levels of organization in a multicellular organism. The most basic unit is the cell; groups of similar cells form tissues; groups of different tissues make up organs; groups of organs form organ systems; cells, tissues, organs, and organ systems combine to form a multicellular organism.

The next level of organization in the body is that of the organ. An organ is a group of tissues that constitutes a distinct structural and functional unit. Thus, the heart is an organ composed of all four tissues, whose function is to pump blood throughout the body. Of course, the heart does not function in isolation; it is part of a system composed of blood and blood vessels as well. The highest level of body organization, then, is that of the organ system.

The body includes nine major organ systems, each composed of various organs and tissues that work together as a functional unit. The chief constituents and prime functions of each system are summarized below. (1) The integumentary system, composed of the skin and associated structures, protects the body from invasion by harmful microorganisms and chemicals; it also prevents water loss from the body. (2) The musculoskeletal system (also referred to separately as the muscle system and the skeletal system), composed of the skeletal muscles and bones (with about 206 of the latter in adults), moves the body and protectively houses its internal organs. (3) The respiratory system, composed of the breathing passages, lungs, and muscles of respiration, obtains from the air the oxygen necessary for cellular metabolism; it also returns to the air the carbon dioxide that forms as a waste product of such metabolism. (4) The circulatory system, composed of the heart, blood, and blood vessels, circulates a transport fluid throughout the body, providing the cells with a steady supply of oxygen and nutrients and carrying away waste products such as carbon dioxide and toxic nitrogen compounds. (5) The digestive system, composed of the mouth, esophagus, stomach, and intestines, breaks down food into usable substances (nutrients), which are then absorbed from the blood or lymph; this system also eliminates the unusable or excess portion of the food as fecal matter. (6) The excretory system, composed of the kidneys, ureters, urinary bladder, and urethra, removes toxic nitrogen compounds and other wastes from the blood. (7) The nervous system, composed of the sensory organs, brain, spinal cord, and nerves, transmits, integrates, and analyzes sensory information and carries impulses to effect the appropriate muscular or glandular responses. (8) The endocrine system, composed of the hormone-secreting glands and tissues, provides a chemical communications network for coordinating various body processes. (9) The reproductive system, composed of the male or female sex organs, enables reproduction and thereby ensures the continuation of the species.

Basic Form and Development

In general structure, the human body follows a plan that can be described as a cylinder enclosing two tubes and a rod. This body plan is most clearly evident in the embryo; by birth, the plan is apparent only in the trunk region—i.e., in the thorax and abdomen.

The body wall forms the cylinder. The two tubes are the ventrally located alimentary canal (i.e., the digestive tract) and the dorsally located neural tube (i.e., the spinal cord). Between the tubes lies the rod—the notochord in the embryo, which becomes the vertebral column prior to birth. (The terms dorsal and ventral refer respectively to the back and the front, or belly, of an animal).

Within the embryo, the essential body parts are: (1) the outer enclosing epidermal membrane (in the embryo called ectoderm); (2) the dorsal neural tube; (3) the supporting notochord; (4) the ventral alimentary tube, which becomes the lining of the stomach and intestine (in the embryo called endoderm); (5) the intermediate mass (in the embryo called mesoderm); and (6) a rather fluid tissue that fills the interspaces, derived from the mesoderm and in the embryo called mesenchyme. Everything in the body derives from one of these six embryonic parts.

The mesoderm constitutes a considerable pad of tissue on each side of the embryo, extending all the way from the back to the front sides of the body wall. It is hollow, for a cleftlike space appears in it on each side. These are the right and left body cavities. In the dorsal part of the body they are temporary; in the ventral part they become permanent, forming the two pleural cavities, which house the lungs; the peritoneal cavity, which contains the abdominal organs; and the pericardial cavity, which encloses the heart. The dorsal part of the mesoderm becomes separated from the ventral mesoderm and divides itself into serial parts like a row of blocks, 31 on each side. These mesodermal segments grow in all directions toward the epidermal membrane. They form bones, muscles, and the deeper, leathery part of the skin. Dorsally they form bony arches protecting the spinal cord, and ventrally the ribs protecting the alimentary canal and heart. Thus they form the body wall and the limbs—much the weightier part of the body. They give the segmental character to the body wall in neck and trunk, and, following their lead, the spinal cord becomes correspondingly segmented. The ventral mesoderm is not so extensive; it remains near the alimentary tube and becomes the continuous muscle layer of the stomach and intestine. It also forms the lining of the body cavities, the smooth, shining, slippery pleura and peritoneum. The mesenchyme forms blood and lymph vessels, the heart, and the loose cells of connective tissues.

The neural tube itself is formed from the ectoderm at a very early stage. Anteriorly (i.e., toward the head) it extends above the open end of the cylinder and is enlarged to form the brain. It is not in immediate contact with the epidermis, for the dorsal mesoderm grows up around it and around the roots of the cranial nerves as a covering, separating the brain from the epidermis. Posteriorly the neural tube terminates in the adult opposite the first lumbar vertebra.

If the cylindrical body wall is followed headward, it is found to terminate ventrally as the tongue, dorsally in the skull around the brain, ears, and eyes. There is a considerable interval between eyes and tongue. This is occupied partly by a deep depression of the epidermis between them, which dips in to join the alimentary tube (lining of the mouth). Posteriorly the ventral body wall joins the dorsal at the tailbone (coccyx), thus terminating the body cavities.

Headward, the alimentary tube extends up in front of the notochord and projects above the upper part of the body wall (tongue) and in front of and below the brain to join the epidermal depression. From the epidermal depression are formed the teeth and most of the mouth lining; from the upper end of the alimentary canal are formed the pharynx, larynx, trachea, and lungs. The alimentary canal at its tail end splits longitudinally into two tubes—an anterior and a posterior. The anterior tube becomes the bladder, urethra, and, in the female, the lining of the vagina, where it joins a depression of the ectoderm. The posterior (dorsal) tube becomes the rectum and ends just in front of the coccyx by joining another ectodermal depression (the anus).

Human Physiological Systems

Physiology is the study of function in living matter; it attempts to explain the physical and chemical factors that are responsible for the origin, development, and progression of life. In human physiology we attempt to explain the events (chemical and electrical) that occur in the body which allow us to exist under a wide variety of conditions.

- Cells as the basic living unit of the body - The basic living unit of the body is the cell. Organs and tissues are actually Assemblies of many different cells. They are held together by supporting structures (tissue, bone, etc.) and work to provide a uniform or greater purpose. Each type of cell is specially adapted to perform its specific function. For instance, the red blood cells are specifically designed to carry oxygen from the lungs to the tissues in the body.

Even though cells may have difference, in some basic ways they are alike. For example:

- Cells are built with cell walls, which is like a skin that separates the fluid inside the cell separate from the fluid outside the cell. These walls are not solid; they have pores which allow substances (like nutrients) to pass in and waste products to escape out.
- Each cell requires nutrition (food) to stay alive; they use almost the same types of nutrients to sustain life; the methods of changing these nutrients into energy is the same; and, almost all cells have the ability to reproduce.
- Cells are automatons (they work automatically) that are capable of living, growing, and providing their special functions so long as the body provides the proper amounts of oxygen, glucose (sugar), electrolytes (electrically charged elements), amino acids, and fatty substances.
- Fluid - Over half of the human body is fluid. There is the fluid which is inside the cells and that is called intracellular fluid; and, there is the fluid which is outside of the cells and that is called the extra cellular fluid.

Intracellular fluid is much the same from one cell to the other but is different from extra cellular fluid in that it contains larger amounts of minerals such as potassium, magnesium, and phosphate ions. Ions are particles that have an electronic charge to them; the charge may be positive (+) or negative (-).

Extra cellular fluid contains large amounts of sodium, chloride, and bicarbonate ions. In addition, the extra cellular fluid carries nutrients (oxygen, glucose, fatty acids, and amino acids) the cells and carries waste (carbon dioxide and excretory products) away from the cells. The extra cellular fluid is in constant motion throughout the body and in its motion into and out of the cells. Therefore, all cells live in essentially the same environment.

The chemical difference between the intracellular fluid and extra cellular fluid establishes a concentration and electronic charge difference which works to move nutrients into the cell, waste out, and in brain cells facilitates communications.

A group of cells may organize into tissue, which means they are connected and work together to perform a similar function. Tissues may be organized into an organ. An organ is a group of tissues that perform a specific function or group of functions. Frequently the tissue is specific for that organ's function—heart muscle tissue is different from brain or liver tissue, for example.

- The major systems - The body has a number of systems of organsestablished to carry out the tasks essential to the functioning and survival of the body. For the most part, it is important for these systems to operate in harmony with each other. This harmony is sometimes called homeostasis. The term homeostasisis used by physiologists to mean the maintenance of steady, consistent conditions (usually referring to the body's internal environment). Essentially all the organs and tissues of the body function to help maintain homeostasis (a stable, internal condition). For example, the lungs provide new oxygen and eliminate old carbon dioxide at rates that are consistent with the body's needs.
- The Fluid Transport System - Extra cellular fluid is transported to all parts of the body in two different stages:

The first stage is the movement of blood around the body via the circulatory system. Essential to this stage is the action of the heart. The heart is actually two separate pumps, one which propels blood through the lungs and the other which propels blood throughout the rest of the body (blood usually moves through the entire body system an average of once every minute when a person is at rest and 5 times each minute when the person is extremely active). Blood pumped through the lungs is essential to picking up oxygen for transport to other parts of the body.

The second stage involves the movement of blood in and out of the cells of the body. Blood and fluids going into cell areas, usually move from larger "pipes"—the veins and arteries—into smaller ones called capillaries. The materials that enter the cell is determined by a number of factors including the size of the material, the porosity (how big are the "doors into" the cell) of the cell membrane, the ionic charge (like how magnets are charged) of the material, and the electrolytic balance in the cell fluids.

- The Respiratory System - Each time the blood passes through the body it also flows through the lungs where it picks up oxygen. Oxygen diffuses (passes) through the membranes of the lung and into the blood in the same way that water, nutrients, and waste products move to and from cells and the blood.

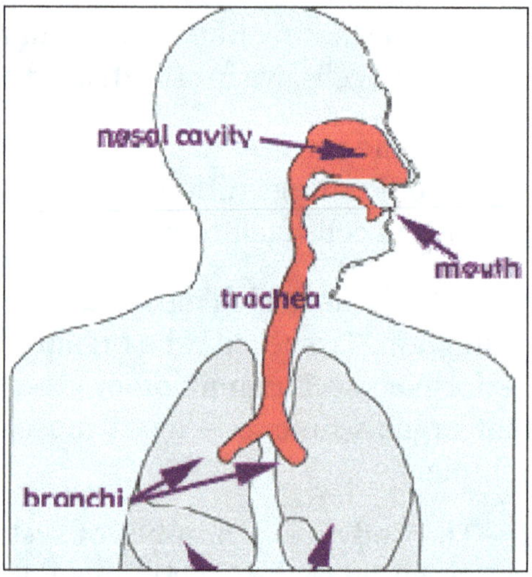

- The Digestive System - The human digestive system is a complex series of organs and glands that processes food. In order to use the food we eat, our body has to break the food down into smaller molecules that it can process; it also has to excrete waste.

Most of the digestive organs (like the stomach and intestines) are tube-like and contain the food as it makes its way through the body. The digestive system is essentially a long, twisting tube that runs from the mouth to the anus, plus a few other organs (like the liver and pancreas) that produce or store digestive chemicals.

An important route for blood is through the walls of the gastrointestinal (GI) organs—especially the small intestine. Blood's job here is to pick up and transport the various dissolved nutrients, including carbohydrates, fatty acids, and amino acids for use by the body. Because not all substances absorbed from the gastrointestinal tract can be used in their absorbed form, they may be transported to the liver where their chemical composition is changed so they are in more useable forms.

The Digestive Process

The Mouth (the start of the process) - The digestive process begins in the mouth. Food is partly broken down by the process of chewing and by the chemical action of salivary enzymes (these enzymes are produced by the salivary glands and break down starches into smaller molecules).

The esophagus (The way to the stomach) - After being chewed and swallowed, the food enters the esophagus. The esophagus is a long tube that runs from the mouth to the stomach. It uses rhythmic, wave-like muscle movements (called peristalsis) to force food from the throat into the stomach. This muscle movement gives us the ability to eat or drink even when we're upside-down.

In the stomach - The stomach is a large, sack-like organ that churns the food and bathes it in a very strong acid (gastric acid).

Small intestine (finer processing area) - After being in the stomach, food enters the duodenum, the first part of the small intestine. It then enters the final part of the small intestine. In the small intestine, bile (produced in the liver and stored in the gall bladder), pancreatic enzymes, and other digestive enzymes produced by the inner wall of the small intestine help in the breakdown of food.

Large intestine (a final squeeze for nutrients) - After passing through the small intestine, food passes into the large intestine. In the large intestine, some of the water and electrolytes (chemicals like sodium) are removed from the food. Many bacteria like microbes in the large intestine help in the digestion process. Food then travels upward in the ascending colon. The food travels across the abdomen in the transverse colon, goes back down the other side of the body in the descending colon, and then through the sigmoid colon.

The end of the process – From the small intestine, food that has not been digested (and some water) travels to the large intestine through a valve that prevents food from returning to the small intestine. By the time food reaches the large intestine, the work of absorbing nutrients is nearly finished. The large intestine's main function is to remove water from the undigested matter and form solid waste that can be excreted.

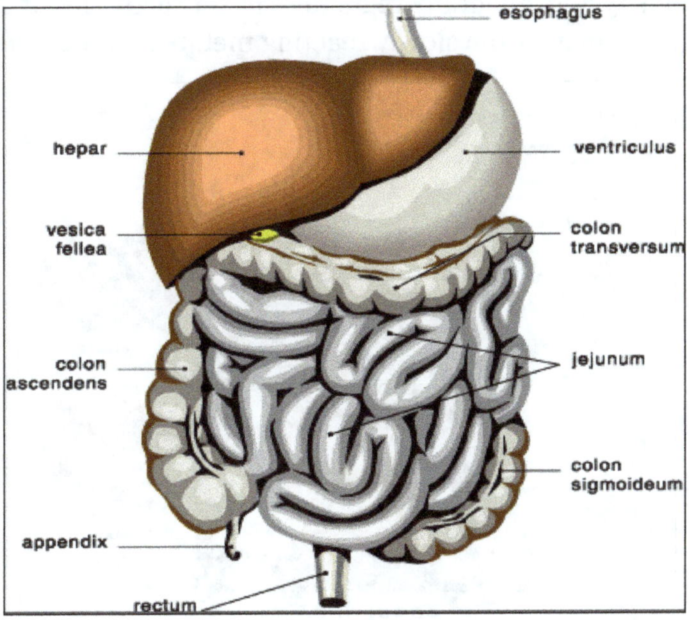

The liver (located under the ribcage in the right upper part of the abdomen), the gallbladder (hidden just below the liver), and the pancreas(beneath the stomach) are not part of the GI system, but these organs are still important for healthy digestion.

The pancreas produces enzymes that help digest proteins, fats, and carbohydrates. It also makes a substance that neutralizes stomach acid. The liver produces bile, which helps the body absorb fat. Bile is stored in the gallbladder until it is needed. These enzymes and bile travel through special channels (called ducts) directly into the small intestine, where they help to break down food.

The liver also plays a major role in the handling and processing of nutrients. These nutrients are carried to the liver in the blood from the small intestine.

- The Musculoskeletal System - Getting the body to move to the right place at the right time is extremely important to survival. Without this system, the ability to get food and escape enemies would be greatly, if not fatally, hindered.
- The Endocrine (hormone) System - Located in the body are eight major endocrine or hormone producing glands. Hormones are transported in the extra cellular fluids to all parts of the body to help regulate functioning. For instance, thyroid hormone increases the rate of almost all chemical reactions in all cells. In this way thyroid hormone helps to set the tempo of bodily activities. Likewise:
    - Insulin controls glucose (sugar) metabolism.
    - Adrenal hormones control many stress reactions in the body.
    - Testosterone and estrogen influence sexual drive.

Whereas the nervous system generally regulates "faster" activities of the body, the hormone system regulates mainly the slowly reacting metabolic functions.

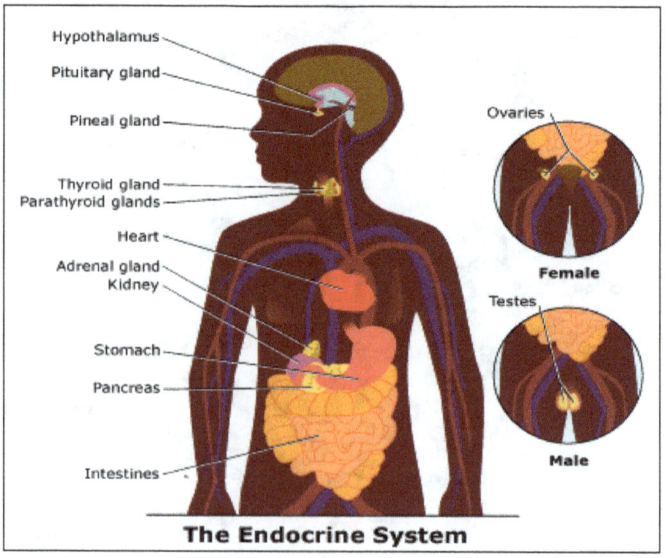

The Endocrine System

The foundations of the endocrine system are the hormones and glands. As the body's chemical messengers, hormones transfer information and instructions from one set of cells to another. Although many different hormones circulate throughout the bloodstream, each one affects only the cells that are genetically programmed to receive and respond to its message. Hormone levels can be influenced by factors such as stress, infection, and changes in the balance of fluid and minerals in blood.

A gland is a group of cells that produces and secretes, or gives off, chemicals. A gland selects and removes materials from the blood, processes them, and secretes the finished chemical product for use somewhere in the body. Endocrine glands release more than 20 major hormones directly into the bloodstream where they can be transported to cells in other parts of the body.

- The "Waste Removal" System - Some other systems like the respiratory and GI systems play key roles in the removal of waste from the body. At the same time that blood picks up oxygen in the lungs, carbon dioxide is released from the blood so it can be eliminated as breath (Carbon dioxide is the most common "end product" of metabolism).

A key organ in the waste removal system is the kidney (or kidneys, because we have two). Passage of blood through the kidneys removes most of the waste and excess water and electrolytes from the body. The kidneys perform their function by first filtering large quantities of plasma (part of the blood which contains high amounts of proteins)—substances that are needed by the body (glucose, amino acids, necessary water and electrolytes) are reabsorbed into the blood. The remaining elements pass through the renal (kidney) tubes into the urine.

- The Nervous System - The nervous system can be divided into several connected systems that function together. The Central Nervous Systemand the Peripheral Nervous System.

The Central Nervous System (CNS) is comprised of the brain and the spinal cord. The average adult human brain weighs approximately 3 pounds. The brain contains about 100 billion nerve cells (neurons) and trillions of "support cells" called glia. The spinal cord is the collection of bones (back bone) that houses the spinal cord.

The Brain - The brain is involved in everything you do, how you think, how you feel, how you act, and how well you get along with other people. When your brain works right, you work right; when your brain doesn't work right, it is very hard to do your best. There are things which hurt our brains, such as injuries, pollution (such as taking drugs), poor nutrition, and excessive stress.

Basic Organization of the Brain - In general terms, the brain can be separated into three main systems:

Old Brain - Represented by the upper spinal chord to the hypothalamus. Primary functions include system arousal level, hormonal control of many basic body survival functions (digestion, breathing, temperature regulation, blood pressure), and a communications network.

Limbic System (middle-aged brain) - Represented by areas that focus on pleasure-reward and emotions. This part of the brain is also important as an integrator of sensory information received to the body and a processor of that information, selecting what is important to pay attention to and take action toward.

Cortex (new-aged brain) - Representing areas important in reasoning, higher level decision making, planning, organizing and sequencing behavior.

All of these tasks are coordinated, controlled and regulated by an organ that is about the size of a small head of cauliflower.

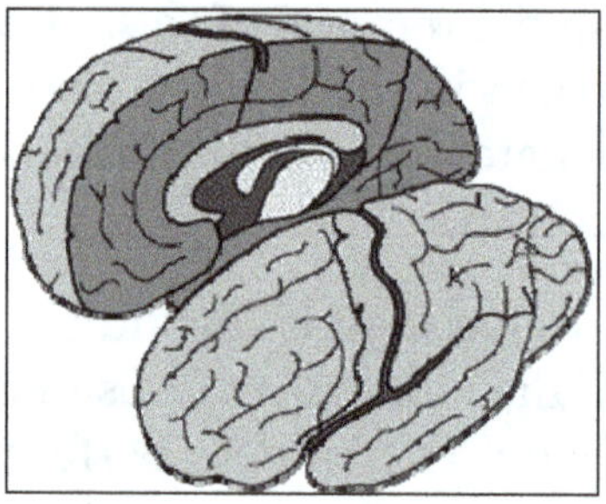

From a top view, notice how the brain is divided into two halves, called hemispheres. Each hemisphere communicates with the other through the corpus callosum, a bundle of nerve fibers.

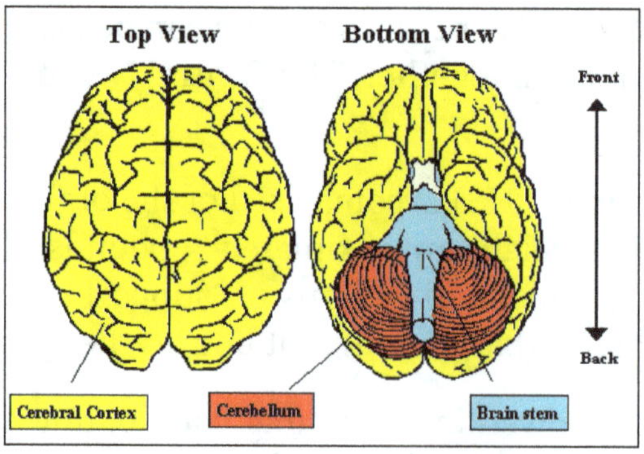

Brain Structures

Cerebral Cortex

Functions:

- Thought,
- Voluntary movement,

- Language,
- Reasoning,
- Perception.

This is because the cortex is a sheet of tissue that makes up the outer layer of the brain. The thickness of the cerebral cortex varies from 2 to 6 mm. The right and left sides of the cerebral cortex are connected by a thick band of nerve fibers called the "corpus callosum." In higher mammals such as humans, the cerebral cortex looks like it has many bumps and grooves. A bump or bulge on the cortex is called a gyrus (the plural of the word gyrus is "gyri") and a groove is called a sulcus (the plural of the word sulcus is "sulci"). Lower mammals, such as rats and mice, have very few gyri and sulci.

Cerebellum

Functions:

- Movement,
- Balance,
- Posture.

The cerebellum is located behind the brain stem. In some ways, the cerebellum is similar to the cerebral cortex: the cerebellum is divided into hemispheres and has a cortex that surrounds these hemispheres.

Brain Stem

Functions:

- Breathing,
- Heart Rate,
- Blood Pressure.

The brain stem is a general term for the area of the brain between the thalamus and spinal cord. Structures within the brain stem include the medulla, pons, tectum, reticular formation and tegmentum. Some of these areas are responsible for the most basic functions of life such as breathing, heart rate and blood pressure.

Hypothalamus

Functions:

- Body Temperature,
- Emotions,

- Hunger,
- Thirst,
- Circadian Rhythms.

The hypothalamus is composed of several different areas and is located at the base of the brain. Although it is the size of only a pea (about 1/300 of the total brain weight), the hypothalamus is responsible for some very important functions. One important function of the hypothalamus is the control of body temperature. The hypothalamus acts as a "thermostat" by sensing changes in body temperature and then sending signals to adjust the temperature. For example, if you are too hot, the hypothalamus detects this and then sends a signal to expand the capillaries in your skin. This causes blood to be cooled faster. The hypothalamus also controls the pituitary.

Thalamus

Functions:

- Sensory processing,
- Movement.

The thalamus receives sensory information and relays this information to the cerebral cortex. The cerebral cortex also sends information to the thalamus which then transmits this information to other areas of the brain and spinal cord.

Limbic System

Functions:

- Emotions.

The limbic system (or the limbic areas) is a group of structures that includes the amygdala, the hippocampus, basal ganglia, ventral tegmental area, and cingulate. These areas are important for controlling the emotional response to a given situation. The hippocampus is also important for memory.

Hippocampus

Functions:

- Learning,
- Memory.

The hippocampus is one part of the limbic system that is important for memory and learning.

Basal Ganglia

Functions:

- Movement.

The basal ganglia are a group of structures, including the globus pallidus, caudate nucleus, subthalamic nucleus, putamen and substantia nigra, that are important in coordinating movement.

Midbrain

Functions:

- Vision,
- Audition,
- Eye Movement,
- Body Movement.

The midbrain includes structures such as the superior and inferior colliculi and red nucleus. There are several other areas also in the midbrain.

Here is where some of these Brain areas are located:

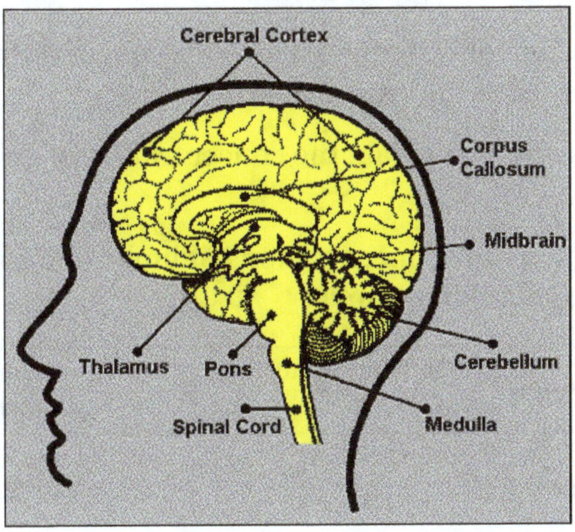

The brain is "wired" with a network of structural neural connections. These connections are not "hard-wired" like in a computer. With some limits, the brains nerve cells (neurons) are able to flexibly change connectivity as the individual's activity demands. This neural flexibility is called plasticity. In much of the brain, the connections are made between neurons that connect the sensory inputs and motor outputs with centers in the various lobes of the cortex. There are also connections between these cortical centers and other parts of the brain.

II. Spinal Cord- The spinal cord is a primary pathway for sensory information.

The spinal cord allows for sensory information than auditory or visual to flow from the body to the brain and for the responses from the brain to transmit back to the body. The spinal cord is also a primary pathway for the autonomic nervous system. The autonomic nervous system is that portion of the nervous system that controls visceral functions of the body. This system helps to control arterial pressure, gastrointestinal motility and secretion, urinary output, sweating, body temperature, and many other activities. The autonomic impulses are transmitted to the body through two major subdivisions called the sympathetic and parasympathetic systems.

Sympathetic - Sometimes called the “fight or flight” response, it is the readiness response of the body, mediated by a neurohormone (messenger) called acetylcholine (nerves that work with acetylcholine are called, cholinergic).

Parsympathetic - Called the “feed or breed” response, it is the relaxation response of the body, mediated by the neurohormone called norepinephrine (nerves that work with norepinephrine are called, adrenergic).

Organizing and orchestrating many of the body’s activities are literally thousands of control systems. Some of these control systems work to control intracellular functions; others operate within the organs to control functions of the individual parts of the organs; others operate throughout the entire body to control the interrelationships between different organs. Some examples include:

- The respiratory control system regulates the concentration of carbon dioxide in the extra cellular fluids and stimulates breathing;
- The liver and pancreas regulate the concentration of glucose in the extra cellular fluids;
- The kidneys regulate the concentrations of important ions like sodium and potassium in the extra cellular fluids.

Organ	Sympathetic Stimulation	Parasympathetic Stimulation
Eye: Pupil	Dilated	Contracted
Glands: Nasal/Lacrimal/ Gastric/Submaxillary/ Pancreatic	Vasoconstriction	Stimulation with secretions containing many enzymes
Sweat Glands	Copious sweating (cholinergic)	None
Heart: Muscle	Increased rate and force of beat	Slower rate and decreased force
Lungs- bronchi Blood vessels	Dilated Mildly constricted	None Increased peristalsis and tone
Gut: lumen Sphincter	Decreased peristalsis and tone Increased tone	Increased peristalsis and tone Decreased tone

Liver	Glucose released	none
Gall bladder and bile ducts	Inhibitcd	Excited
Kidney	Decreased output	None
Systemic Blood vessels: *abdominal *muscle *skin	Constricted Constricted Constricted/dilated Constricted/dilated	Dilated
Blood coagulation and glucose	Increased	None
Basal Metabolism	Increased	None
Mental activity	Increased	None
Piloerector muscles	Stimulated	None

III. Nerve Cells - Part of the nervous system is in the brain. The basic unit of the nervous system is the nerve cell, or neuron. Neurons transmit information. Within the body, the nerves branch out like telephone wires from an exchange. They run to every part of the body, from the bottom of the feet to the top of the head and from just below the skin to the inner organs.

Neurons are found in the central nervous system, which includes your brain and spinal cord, and the peripheral nervous system, which includes all the nerves that reach your body's extremities. Neurons can be divided into three different categories:

- Sensory (or afferent) neurons carry messages to the brain and spinal cord.
- Motor (or efferent) neurons carry messages away from the brain and spinal cord. They tell muscles to contract or relax and to activate glands.
- Interneurons send messages between nerve cells within the brain, spinal cord, and the periphery.

Neuron Structure

Your brain is made of approximately 100-billion nerve cells, called neurons. Neurons have the amazing ability to gather and transmit electrochemical signals - they are something like the gates and wires in a computer. Neurons vary greatly in size and shape. The longest neurons are those that extend down the leg as part of the sciatic nerve. The average nerve running from the base of the spine to the tip of a toe is about 3 feet long, but many other axons are only a fraction of an inch in length. Even though the sizes of neurons vary, all nerve cells have a similar structure.

Neurons have three basic parts:

- Cell body - This main part has all of the necessary components of the cell, such as the nucleus (contains DNA), endoplasmic reticulum and ribosomes (for building proteins) and mitochondria (for making energy). If the cell body dies, the neuron dies.

- Axon - This long, cable-like projection of the cell carries the electrochemical message (nerve impulse or action potential) along the length of the cell.
    - Depending upon the type of neuron, axons can be covered with a thin layer of myelin, like an insulated electrical wire. Myelin is made of fat, and it helps to speed transmission of a nerve impulse down a long axon. Myelinated (fat coated) neurons are usually found in the peripheral nerves (they are sensory and motor neurons), while non-myelinated neurons are found in the brain and spinal cord.
- Dendrites or nerve endings - These small, branch-like projections of the cell make connections to other cells and allow the neuron to talk with other cells or get information from the environment. Dendrites can be located on one or both ends of the cell.

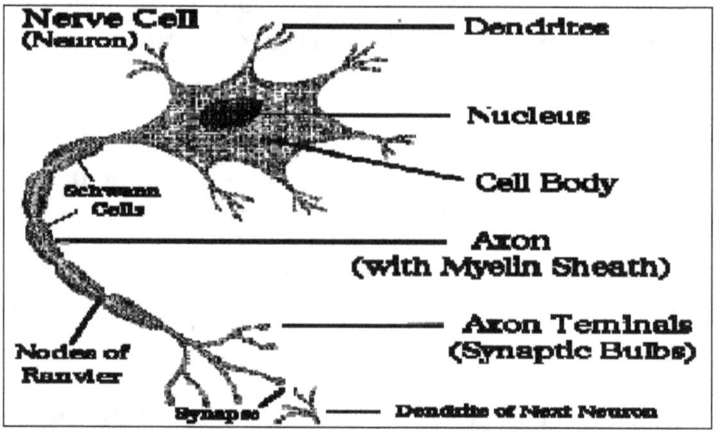

Basic Neuron Types

Neurons come in many sizes. For example, a single sensory neuron from your fingertip has an axon that extends the length of your arm, while neurons within the brain may extend only a few millimeters. Neurons have different shapes depending on what they do. Motor neurons that control muscle contractions have a cell body on one end, a long axon in the middle and dendrites on the other end; sensory neurons have dendrites on both ends, connected by a long axon with a cell body in the middle.

Neurons also vary with respect to their functions:

- Sensory neurons carry signals from the outer parts of your body (periphery) into the central nervous system.
- Motor neurons (motoneurons) carry signals from the central nervous system to the outer parts (muscles, skin, glands) of your body.

- Receptors sense the environment (chemicals, light, sound, touch) and encode this information into electrochemical messages that are transmitted by sensory neurons.
- Interneurons connect various neurons within the brain and spinal cord.

The simplest type of neural pathway is a monosynaptic (single connection) reflex pathway, like the knee-jerk reflex. When the doctor taps the the right spot on your knee with a rubber hammer, receptors send a signal into the spinal cord through a sensory neuron. The sensory neuron passes the message to a motor neuron that controls your leg muscles. Nerve impulses travel down the motor neuron and stimulate the appropriate leg muscle to contract. The response is a muscular jerk that happens quickly and does not involve your brain. Humans have lots of hard-wired reflexes like this, but as tasks become more complex, the pathway "circuitry" gets more complicated and the brain gets involved.

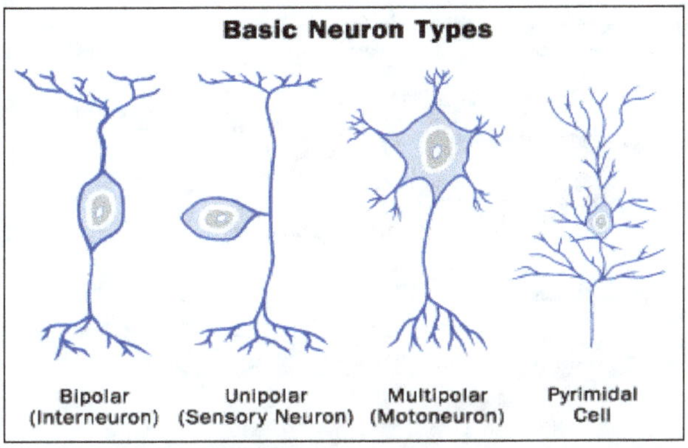

Some types of neurons: Motoneuron, sensory neuron, cortical pyramidal cell.

Skeletal Muscle Physiology

The best known feature of skeletal muscle is its ability to contract and cause movement. Skeletal muscles act not only to produce movement but also to stop movement, such as resisting gravity to maintain posture. Small, constant adjustments of the skeletal muscles are needed to hold a body upright or balanced in any position. Muscles also prevent excess movement of the bones and joints, maintaining skeletal stability and preventing skeletal structure damage or deformation. Joints can become misaligned or dislocated entirely by pulling on the associated bones; muscles work to keep joints stable. Skeletal muscles are located throughout the body at the openings of internal tracts to control the movement of various substances. These muscles allow functions, such as swallowing, urination, and defecation, to be under voluntary control. Skeletal muscles also protect internal organs (particularly abdominal and pelvic organs) by acting as an external barrier or shield to external trauma and by supporting the weight of the organs.

Skeletal muscles contribute to the maintenance of homeostasis in the body by generating heat. Muscle contraction requires energy, and when ATP is broken down, heat is produced. This heat is very noticeable during exercise, when sustained muscle movement causes body temperature to rise, and in cases of extreme cold, when shivering produces random skeletal muscle contractions to generate heat.

Each skeletal muscle is an organ that consists of various integrated tissues. These tissues include the skeletal muscle fibers, blood vessels, nerve fibers, and connective tissue. Each skeletal muscle has three layers of connective tissue (called "mysia") that enclose it and provide structure to the muscle as a whole, and also compartmentalize the muscle fibers within the muscle. Each muscle is wrapped in a sheath of dense, irregular connective tissue called the epimysium, which allows a muscle to contract and move powerfully while maintaining its structural integrity. The epimysium also separates muscle from other tissues and organs in the area, allowing the muscle to move independently.

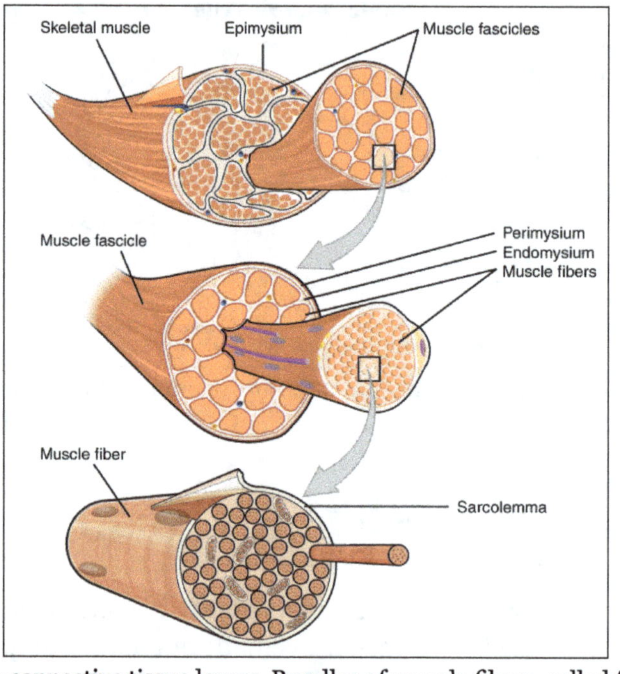

The three connective tissue layers. Bundles of muscle fibers, called fascicles, are covered by the perimysium. Muscle fibers are covered by the endomysium.

Inside each skeletal muscle, muscle fibers are organized into individual bundles, each called a fascicle, by a middle layer of connective tissue called the perimysium. This fascicular organization is common in muscles of the limbs; it allows the nervous system to trigger a specific movement of a muscle by activating a subset of muscle fibers within a bundle, or fascicle of the muscle. Inside each fascicle, each muscle fiber is encased in a thin connective tissue layer of collagen and reticular fibers called the endomysium. The endomysium contains the extracellular fluid and nutrients to support the muscle fiber. These nutrients are supplied via blood to the muscle tissue.

In skeletal muscles that work with tendons to pull on bones, the collagen in the three tissue layers (the mysia) intertwines with the collagen of a tendon. At the other end of the tendon, it fuses with the periosteum coating the bone. The tension created by contraction of the muscle fibers is then transferred though the mysia, to the tendon, and then to the periosteum to pull on the bone for movement of the skeleton. In other places, the mysia may fuse with a broad, tendon-like sheet called an aponeurosis, or to fascia, the connective tissue between skin and bones. The broad sheet of connective tissue in the lower back that the latissimus dorsi muscles (the "lats") fuse into is an example of an aponeurosis.

Every skeletal muscle is also richly supplied by blood vessels for nourishment, oxygen delivery, and waste removal. In addition, every muscle fiber in a skeletal muscle is supplied by the axon branch of a somatic motor neuron, which signals the fiber to contract. Unlike cardiac and smooth muscle, the only way to functionally contract a skeletal muscle is through signaling from the nervous system.

Skeletal Muscle Fibers

Because skeletal muscle cells are long and cylindrical, they are commonly referred to as muscle fibers. Skeletal muscle fibers can be quite large for human cells, with diameters up to 100 μm and lengths up to 30 cm (11.8 in) in the Sartorius of the upper leg. During early development, embryonic myoblasts, each with its own nucleus, fuse with up to hundreds of other myoblasts to form the multinucleated skeletal muscle fibers. Multiple nuclei mean multiple copies of genes, permitting the production of the large amounts of proteins and enzymes needed for muscle contraction.

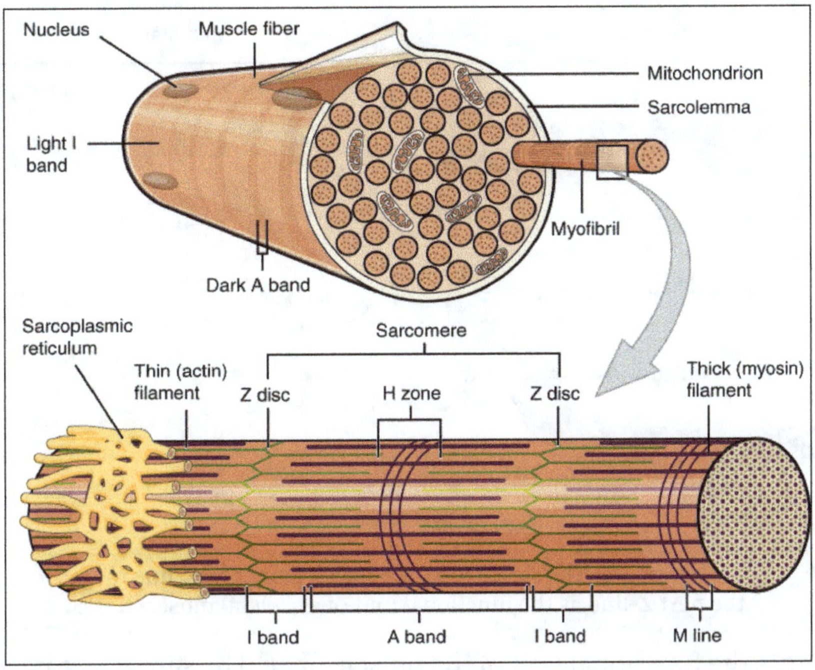

Muscle Fiber: A skeletal muscle fiber is surrounded by a plasma membrane called the sarcolemma, which contains sarcoplasm, the cytoplasm of muscle cells. A muscle fiber is composed of many fibrils, which give the cell its striated appearance.

Some other terminology associated with muscle fibers is rooted in the Greek sarco, which means "flesh." The plasma membrane of muscle fibers is called the sarcolemma, the cytoplasm is referred to as sarcoplasm, and the specialized smooth endoplasmic reticulum, which stores, releases, and retrieves calcium ions (Ca^{++}) is called the sarcoplasmic reticulum (SR). The functional unit of a skeletal muscle fiber is the sarcomere, a highly organized arrangement of the contractile myofilaments actin (thin filament) and myosin (thick filament), along with other support proteins.

Sarcomere

The striated appearance of skeletal muscle fibers is due to the arrangement of the myofilaments of actin and myosin in sequential order from one end of the muscle fiber to the other. Each packet of these microfilaments and their regulatory proteins, troponin and tropomyosin (along with other proteins) is called a sarcomere.

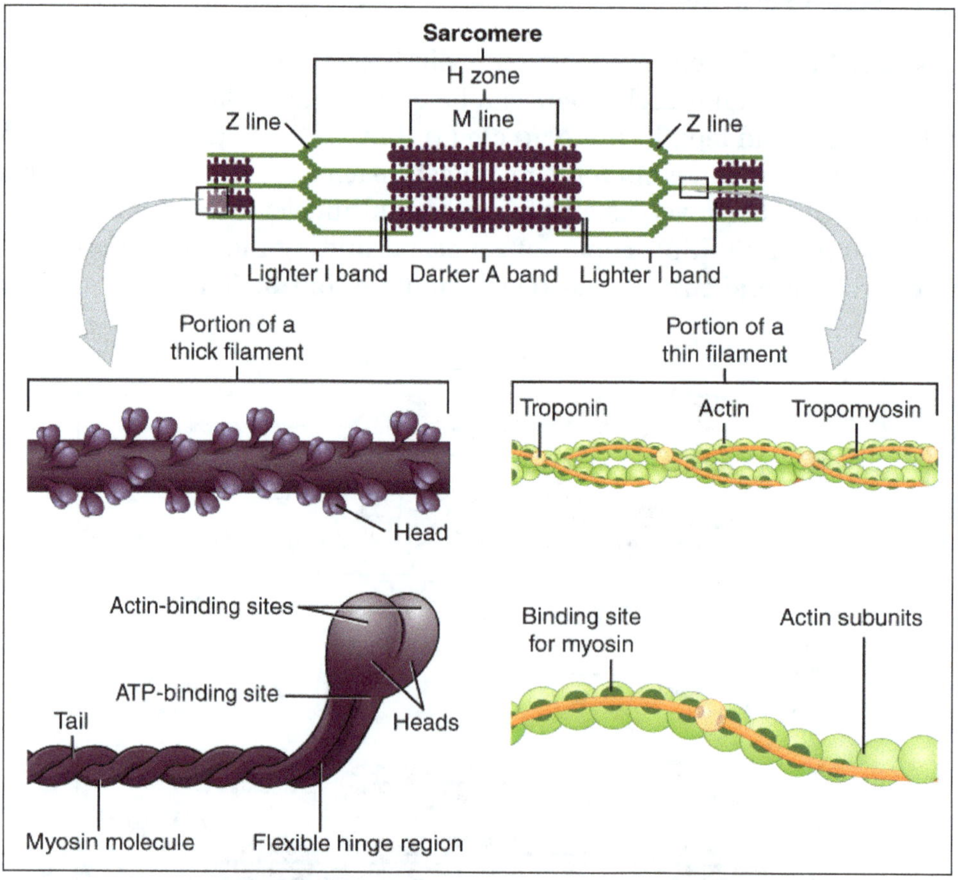

Sarcomere: The sarcomere, the region from one Z-line to the next Z-line, is the functional unit of a skeletal muscle fiber.

The sarcomere is the functional unit of the muscle fiber. The sarcomere itself is bundled within the myofibril that runs the entire length of the muscle fiber and attaches to the sarcolemma at its end. As myofibrils contract, the entire muscle cell contracts. Because myofibrils are only approximately 1.2 μm in diameter, hundreds to thousands (each with thousands of sarcomeres) can be found inside one muscle fiber. Each sarcomere is approximately 2 μm in length with a three-dimensional cylinder-like arrangement and is bordered by structures called Z-discs (also called Z-lines, because pictures are two-dimensional), to which the actin myofilaments are anchored. Because the actin and its troponin-tropomyosin complex (projecting from the Z-discs toward the center of the sarcomere) form strands that are thinner than the myosin, it is called the thin filament of the sarcomere. Likewise, because the myosin strands and their multiple heads (projecting from the center of the sarcomere, toward but not all to way to, the Z-discs) have more mass and are thicker, they are called the thick filament of the sarcomere.

Neuromuscular Junction

Another specialization of the skeletal muscle is the site where a motor neuron's terminal meets the muscle fiber—called the neuromuscular junction (NMJ). This is where the muscle fiber first responds to signaling by the motor neuron. Every skeletal muscle fiber in every skeletal muscle is innervated by a motor neuron at the NMJ. Excitation signals from the neuron are the only way to functionally activate the fiber to contract.

Excitation-contraction Coupling

All living cells have membrane potentials, or electrical gradients across their membranes. The inside of the membrane is usually around -60 to -90 mV, relative to the outside. This is referred to as a cell's membrane potential. Neurons and muscle cells can use their membrane potentials to generate electrical signals. They do this by controlling the movement of charged particles, called ions, across their membranes to create electrical currents. This is achieved by opening and closing specialized proteins in the membrane called ion channels. Although the currents generated by ions moving through these channel proteins are very small, they form the basis of both neural signaling and muscle contraction.

Both neurons and skeletal muscle cells are electrically excitable, meaning that they are able to generate action potentials. An action potential is a special type of electrical signal that can travel along a cell membrane as a wave. This allows a signal to be transmitted quickly and faithfully over long distances.

Although the term excitation-contraction coupling confuses or scares some students, it comes down to this: for a skeletal muscle fiber to contract, its membrane must first be "excited"—in other words, it must be stimulated to fire an action potential. The muscle fiber action potential, which sweeps along the sarcolemma as a wave, is "coupled" to the actual contraction through the release of calcium ions (Ca^{++}) from the SR. Once released, the Ca^{++} interacts with the shielding proteins, forcing them to move aside so that the actin-binding sites are available for attachment by myosin heads. The myosin then pulls the actin filaments toward the center, shortening the muscle fiber.

In skeletal muscle, this sequence begins with signals from the somatic motor division of the nervous system. In other words, the "excitation" step in skeletal muscles is always triggered by signaling from the nervous system.

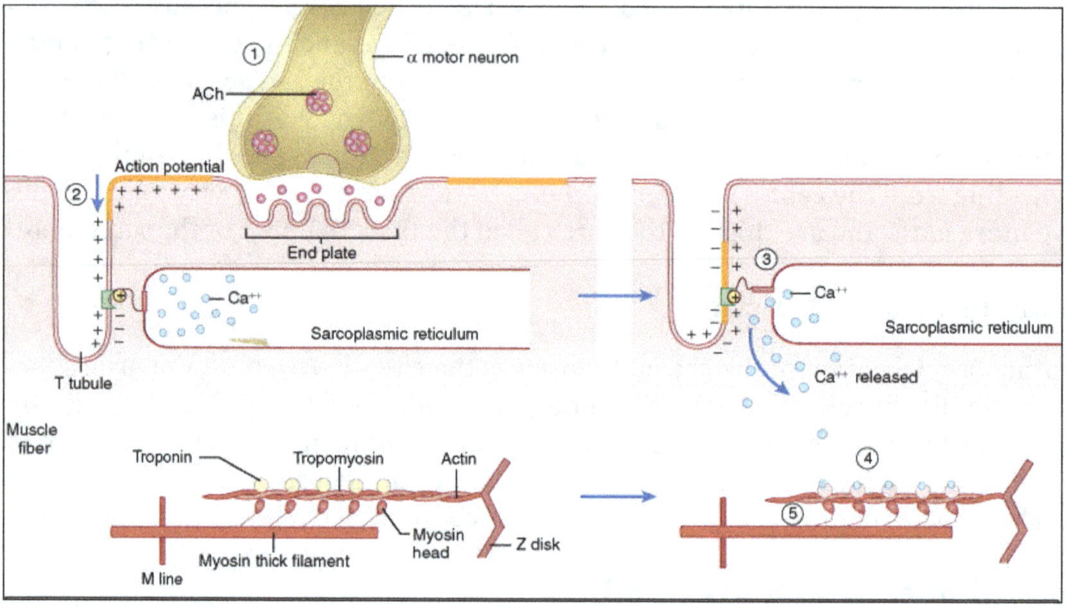

Motor End-Plate and Innervation: At the NMJ, the axon terminal releases ACh. The motor end-plate is the location of the ACh-receptors in the muscle fiber sarcolemma. When ACh molecules are released, they diffuse across a minute space called the synaptic cleft and bind to the receptors.

The motor neurons that tell the skeletal muscle fibers to contract originate in the spinal cord, with a smaller number located in the brainstem for activation of skeletal muscles of the face, head, and neck. These neurons have long processes, called axons, which are specialized to transmit action potentials long distances— in this case, all the way from the spinal cord to the muscle itself (which may be up to three feet away). The axons of multiple neurons bundle together to form nerves, like wires bundled together in a cable.

Signaling begins when a neuronal action potential travels along the axon of a motor neuron, and then along the individual branches to terminate at the NMJ. At the NMJ, the axon terminal releases a chemical messenger, or neurotransmitter, called acetylcholine (ACh). The ACh molecules diffuse across a minute space called the synaptic cleft and bind to ACh receptors located within the motor end-plate of the sarcolemma on the other side of the synapse. Once ACh binds, a channel in the ACh receptor opens and positively charged ions can pass through into the muscle fiber, causing it to depolarize, meaning that the membrane potential of the muscle fiber becomes less negative (closer to zero).

As the membrane depolarizes, another set of ion channels called voltage-gated sodium channels are triggered to open. Sodium ions enter the muscle fiber, and an action potential rapidly spreads (or "fires") along the entire membrane to initiate excitation-contraction coupling.

Things happen very quickly in the world of excitable membranes (just think about how quickly you can snap your fingers as soon as you decide to do it). Immediately following depolarization of the membrane, it repolarizes, re-establishing the negative membrane potential. Meanwhile, the ACh in the synaptic cleft is degraded by the enzyme acetylcholinesterase (AChE) so that the ACh cannot rebind to a receptor and reopen its channel, which would cause unwanted extended muscle excitation and contraction.

Propagation of an action potential along the sarcolemma is the excitation portion of excitation-contraction coupling. Recall that this excitation actually triggers the release of calcium ions (Ca^{++}) from its storage in the cell's SR. For the action potential to reach the membrane of the SR, there are periodic invaginations in the sarcolemma, called T-tubules ("T" stands for "transverse"). You will recall that the diameter of a muscle fiber can be up to 100 μm, so these T-tubules ensure that the membrane can get close to the SR in the sarcoplasm. The arrangement of a T-tubule with the membranes of SR on either side is called a triad. The triad surrounds the cylindrical structure called a myofibril, which contains actin and myosin.

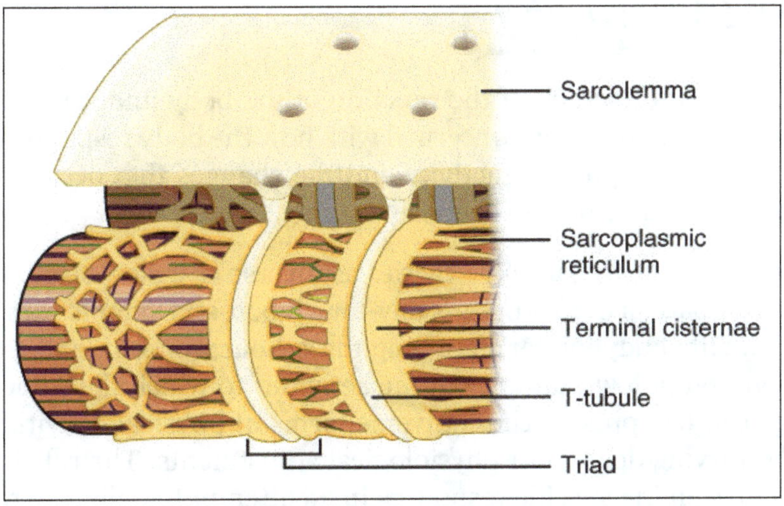

The T-tubule. Narrow T-tubules permit the conduction of electrical impulses. The SR functions to regulate intracellular levels of calcium. Two terminal cisternae (where enlarged SR connects to the T-tubule) and one T-tubule comprise a triad—a "threesome" of membranes, with those of SR on two sides and the T-tubule sandwiched between them.

The T-tubules carry the action potential into the interior of the cell, which triggers the opening of calcium channels in the membrane of the adjacent SR, causing Ca^{++} to diffuse out of the SR and into the sarcoplasm. It is the arrival of Ca^{++} in the sarcoplasm that initiates contraction of the muscle fiber by its contractile units, or sarcomeres.

2

Exercise Physiology, Immunology and Kinesiology

The physiology of physical science is termed as exercise physiology. Biological equilibrium of energy in the human body is called energy balance. The study of immune system is defined as immunology. The study of body movements in all organisms is defined as kinesiology. This chapter closely examines exercise physiology, immunology and kinesiology to provide an extensive understanding of the subject.

Exercise Physiology

Exercise physiology is the study of the function of the body under the stress of acute and chronic exercise. It is equally concerned with how the body responds to the intense demands placed on it by physical activity and the changes that occur in the body as individuals regularly participate in exercise training.

Physical activity takes many forms. Activities as diverse as a slow stroll, raking leaves, a mile run at a fast pace, a dock worker's day-long labor, an Olympic weightlifter's 200 kg snatch lift, an elite bodybuilder's grueling three-hour workout, and a marathoner's 26.2-mile run are but a few examples of the activities to which the principles of exercise physiology can be applied. These diverse forms of physical activities require our bodies to make varying degrees of physiological adjustments. The role of the exercise physiologist is to examine specific responses in an attempt to delineate the alterations made with acute exercise to better understand the chronic adaptations that occur with exercise training.

The term acute refers to the performance of a single bout of exercise. This may take a few seconds (running a 40-yard dash) or many hours (competing in an ultramarathon race). Exercise physiologists investigate how the body makes internal adjustments in the face of massive disruptions to homeostasis occurring with exercise stress.

The study of acute responses represents only half of what is of interest in exercise physiology. Of concern also are the adaptive processes to chronic exercise stress. The term chronic refers to a length of time over which changes take place in different physiological systems during exercise training. These changes, or adaptations, generally can be interpreted as an improvement in the body's function at rest and during submaximal and maximal exercise.

Using the framework of acute responses and chronic adaptations, the exercise physiologist applies the knowledge gained from the basic sciences to problems in exercise physiology, thereby gaining insights into how the body functions during the stress of exercise. This can then be used as a basis for developing the best training practices to enhance athletic performance or improve health, two areas of special interest to the exercise physiologist.

Metabolic and Hemodynamic Continua

The differences in the acute responses and chronic adaptations among physical activities are often astounding. For example, it is possible to classify all exercises, athletic activities, and general physical activities on continua based on the two key physiological perturbations to exercise—*metabolic* and *hemodynamic* responses. In terms of metabolic responses, exercises can range from those that require the anaerobic production of energy in the cell to those that require the aerobic production of energy. In terms of hemodynamic responses, exercises can range from those that impose a volume load on the heart to those that impose a pressure load.

The metabolic continuum illustrates physical activities as energetic events. Activities are placed in a time frame that depicts the duration of the maximal effort during the event. The descriptors power, speed, and endurance are intensity factors with the greatest intensity (and shortage duration) being on the power end of the continuum and the lowest intensity (and longest duration) on the endurance end. Power and speed events are anaerobic, that is, they do not require the production of adenosine triphosphate (ATP) via oxygen metabolism to fuel the event. The further an event moves along the continuum toward the right, the more it relies on oxygen metabolism and the longer will be the duration of the event or exercise. Therefore, endurance events are aerobic, requiring oxygen for the production of ATP.

Track and field events are ideal examples of the use of these descriptors. For instance, the shotput requires all-out effort from the first instance of movement to displace the shot with as much force and distance as possible.

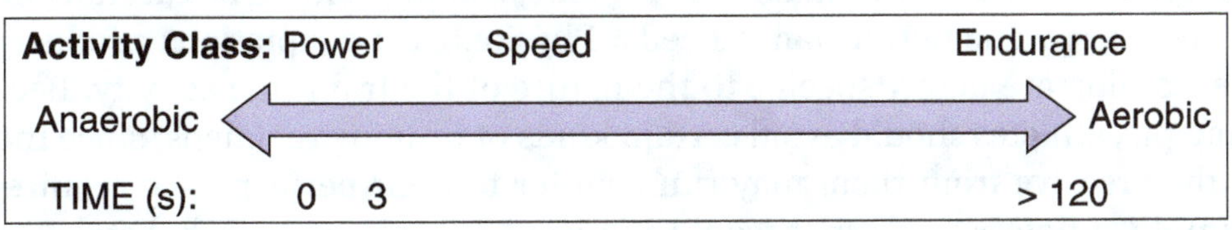

Metabolic continuum.

The event is over in less than 3 seconds. Other examples of power activities are Olympic weightlifting (single, maximal lifts) and running up a short flight of stairs. From an energetics standpoint, the fuel used for events classed in the power category is resting stores of phosphagens, particularly ATP and creatine phosphate (CP).

Speed events require a slightly longer time period. Examples of speed events are sprints

(100 and 200 meters) and longer runs (400 meters). Weightlifting performed as a bodybuilding routine involving many repetitions per bout also qualifies as a speed event since the time frame during which the performer lifts is longer, but not approaching the endurance end of the continuum. Events and exercises of this nature rely on glycogen stores in the muscles to fuel maximal performance of the activity, which results in the production of lactic acid. Lactic acid buildup is what sets the boundary for duration of the maximal effort during speed events.

Endurance events are at the extreme right end of the continuum and are of much longer duration than both power and speed events. However, endurance activities are not very intense, allowing the production of ATP largely through aerobic metabolism. The 1500-meter run and runs of much longer duration are in this category. It must be noted that activities are not mutually exclusive in a metabolic sense; no one activity relies solely on a single energy system.

Sometimes placing an event or activity or sport on the metabolic continuum to determine the main way ATP is supplied to the contracting muscle can be tricky. For example, is soccer play aerobic or anaerobic? What about basketball? The answer to those questions depends on the action of the performer. If the play is of low intensity, as is sometimes the case, aerobic production of ATP predominates. If, however, an athlete steals the ball and there is a fast break to the goal, the anaerobic production of ATP predominates. So how would such an athlete train? The answer is that training should employ a combination of methods to ready the athlete for the various rigors of the sport.

It can be seen then that some activities fall in a "gray" zone with the energy output dependent on both anaerobic and aerobic sources. Generally, the shorter the activity, the greater is the contribution of anaerobic energy production. Conversely, the longer the activity, the greater is the contribution of aerobic energy pro- duction. The type of training program adopted to improve performance in an activity or sport event depends heavily on where the activity falls on the continuum.

An important concept related to the metabolic continuum and the type of exercise training employed is specificity. To maximize benefits, training should be carefully matched to an athlete's specific performance needs. Physiological adaptations produced from exercise training are highly specific to the nature of the train- ing activity. Because of this principle, athletes should avoid certain kinds of training regimens, since the adaptations they receive from them may run counter to their performance requirements. For example, a power performer would not want to train with long distance jogging because the physiological adaptations gained from that form of exercise would tend to weaken his performance in the power event or sport.

Another example is the classic misconception that weight training will produce aerobic or cardiovascular benefits. The reasons why this is false are physiological and biochemical in nature and relate to the fact that specific kinds of adaptations (i.e., the aerobic benefits supposedly produced by weight training) follow only if there is a demand made on the bioenergetic processes and the physiological systems thought to be adapting. Cardiovascular benefits do not follow weight training because weightlifting does not sufficiently engage aero- bic bioenergetic pathways.

Exercise can also be classified on a hemodynamic continuum. The degree to which an activity promotes blood movement (volume load) and the amount of blood pressure produced (pressure load) by the activity are important considerations when attempting to understand acute responses.

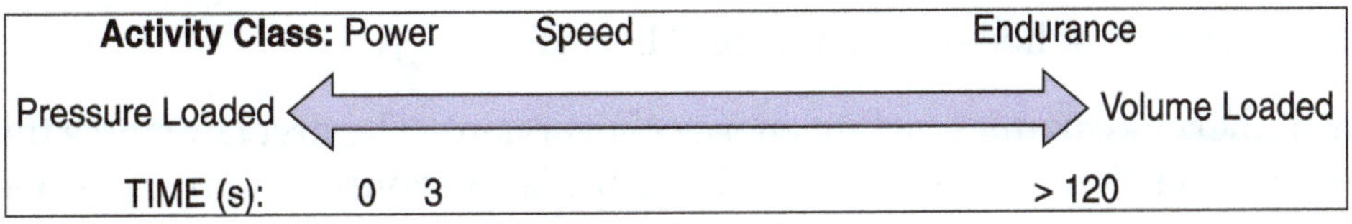

Hemodynamic continuum.

Hemodynamic refers to the circulation of blood and encompass the forces restricting or promoting its circulation. Exercises that promote a great deal of blood movement are the endurance forms. These exercises are also associated with moderate elevations in blood pressure and are classified under the volume load heading. In typical aerobic or endurance exercise, the heart is loaded or stressed by pumping a great deal of blood volume through the circulation. There is a necessary link between aerobic metabolism (the metabolic continuum) and blood flow (the hemodynamic continuum). When an exercise is primarily aerobic, the hemodynamic response is largely one that promotes large blood flow. In contrast, those exercises that restrict blood movement, as in resistance forms (weightlifting), are also the ones that lead to a sharp increase in blood pressure. The heart is said to be pressure loaded in this class of exercise. While resistance exercise promotes moderate increases in blood movement, the amount of blood flow during resistance exercise is still very limited in comparison to volume load exercise. Therefore, pressure load exercises also are said to be largely anaerobic. Weightlifting is a perfect example of a pressure load exercise.

Activities, exercises, and sports events will fall at some point along the continua, but a few can be placed at either extreme. The concept of metabolic and hemodynamic continua is extremely useful in helping the coach or personal trainer design the best exercise training programs for clients. With knowledge of where a sport event or exercise falls on the continua, it becomes a matter of designing an exercise program that stresses train- ing in the time frame of the event. For those sports events that are somewhere in the middle of the metabolic continuum, a mixed training program is needed.

Energy

Understanding energy conversion in the cell is vital for a sound understanding of muscular activity. The most rudimentary understanding of movement can be reduced to the study of the biochemical processes that release bound energy, converting it to free energy that is involved at any moment in all biological processes. Energy is the ability to perform work. Work and energy are directly related; as work increases, so does the transfer of energy from one form to another.

Different forms of energy are important in biological processes. The following are a few examples:

- Skeletal and heart muscle contraction, metabolic processes: Chemical energy.
- Nerve conduction: electrical energy.
- Maintenance of body temperature: Thermal energy.

The laws of thermodynamics dictate energy conversions. The first law states that energy conversions result in no lost energy. This is the law of conservation of energy—energy is neither created nor destroyed, but is converted from one form to another.

The body's bioenergetic systems are part of the thermal processes that govern life on the entire planet, the sun being the ultimate source of energy for life. The massive amount of thermonuclear energy on the sun is released during fusion reactions, which then irradiates the earth where it drives the reactions of photosynthe- sis, the process that makes carbohydrates in plants.

The energy from one reaction (energy releasing—exergonic) is transformed to another form (energy absorbing—endergonic). Exergonic and endergonic reactions are coupled. In the example of photosynthesis radiant energy from fusion reactions (exergonic) on the sun is transformed to chemical energy in the form of carbohydrates (endergonic) on earth. The same coupling of energy-releasing and energy-conserving reactions takes place in our cells with muscle contraction (an endergonic process) being the ultimate outcome.

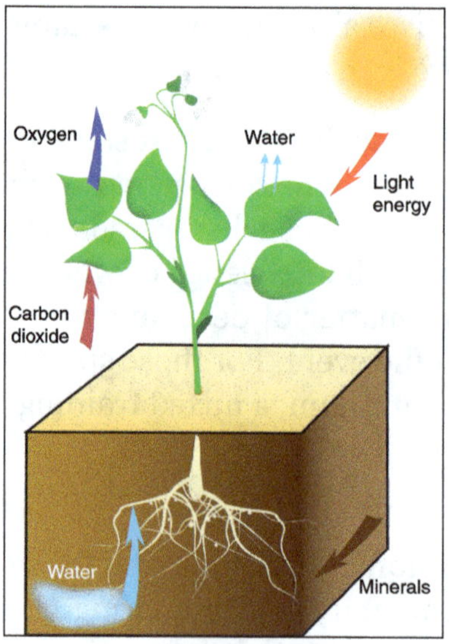

The exergonic process on in the sun is nuclear fusion, which gives off energy in the form of the light and heat. Plants capture this energy and use it to build carbohydrates and other chemical compounds. Since the sun is releasing energy, its reaction is exergonic, and since plants are storing this energy, their reaction is endergonic.

Energy for movement comes from energy-rich nutrients in the form of carbohydrates, fats, and proteins. These three energy nutrients are broken down during digestion to their constituent building-block molecules that enter the body from the digestive tract and are processed by the liver for storage and usage. These building-block molecules are rich in potential energy that is available to be converted to free energy for future muscular work. The energy bound in the building-block molecules, however, cannot be directly used by the contracting muscle. It must first be converted to another chemical form that can then become the direct source of energy for muscle contraction.

Metabolism is the sum of the chemical processes that convert energy from indirect sources (the energy nutrients) to the source that can be used directly to do muscular activity. Another way to state this is that metab- olism is the sum of all catabolic and anabolic reactions. Catabolism is the process of breaking down large energy nutrient molecules to their smaller constituent building blocks. In this process a transfer of energy takes place.

Anabolism is the process whereby smaller biomolecules are built up to larger biomolecules (glucose to glycogen, for example). An input of free energy is necessary to produce these kinds of reactions, making them energy-requiring reactions. For movement to occur, catabolic (energy releasing—exergonic) processes are linked with anabolic (energy trapping—endergonic) processes for the purpose of producing another high- energy product that then becomes the direct donor of free energy for muscular activity. This high-energy compound is ATP.

The subsequent breakdown of ATP releases its bound energy, converting it to free energy, which is then used for all of the energy-requiring processes in our cells, including muscle contraction. How ATP is created in the cell to power muscular activity is one of the major topics in the study of exercise physiology. As we have seen, the processes that produce ATP can proceed by anaerobic or aerobic means. These metabolic pathways are controlled by mechanisms inside the cell that regulate energy storage. All of this activity is precisely inte- grated for the most efficient production of ATP for a given sport activity or exercise.

Anaerobic Production of ATP

ATP can be produced without involving the cellular mechanisms that involve oxygen. The anaerobic production of ATP is a very important means of powering movement and makes possible a greatly expanded repertoire of activities. Table provides examples of activities that are powered by the anaerobic production of ATP divided into power and speed activities. Without the anaerobic production of ATP, activities such as a sprinting or heavy weightlifting would not be possible. What makes power and speed activities possible is the rapid production of ATP in the cell by means of anaerobic metabolic pathways.

Table: Examples of the time course of anaerobic sport events and bodybuilding training.

Activity	Power	Speed	Duration (s)
Weight Training (Olympic Style)	X		< 5
Track and Field Throwing Events	X		< 10
100 m sprint	X		
200 m sprint		X	< 20
Weight Training (Bodybuilding)		X	> 30
400 m run		X	< 45

The phosphagen system is the first and simplest anaerobic metabolic pathway, so named because it uses two important high energy phosphate compounds stored in muscles in small quantities. The release of energy from ATP upon its breakdown causes muscle fibers to shorten (contraction). Every cell in the body contains a quantity of ATP and other high-energy phosphates. These quantities are very small, and because the high energy phosphates cannot be supplied from other areas of the body to the muscle, ATP must be continuously remade in muscle and every other cell. The energy charge of the cell, therefore, is directly related to ATP concentration—low ATP concentration means low energy charge and vice versa. A central role of metabolism is to guarantee that the cell is properly charged by the transfer of bound energy in the form of the energy nutrients to ATP, a process called phosphorylation.

Because anaerobic activities are highly intense, they require a very rapid re-supply of ATP for the rate of muscle contraction, and therefore the activity, to be sustained. Aerobic activities are much less intense, which means ATP production can proceed slowly through the coordinated integration of both cellular and cardiopulmonary system interactions.

To understand these differences more fully, it is important to introduce the concept of metabolic power versus metabolic capacity. A metabolic pathway is powerful if it has the ability to rapidly supply ATP during highly intense activity. Therefore, power relates to the rapidity of the pathway to produce ATP. Capacity, however, refers to the ability to make large quantities of ATP. Power and capacity are inversely related. Metabolic pathways that are the most powerful also have the least capacity, and vice versa. The anaerobic pathways are far more powerful than the aerobic pathways, but have a very limited capacity for ATP production.

ATP is referred to as the energy currency of the cell, because the free energy released from its breakdown powers cellular functions, including muscular contraction. However, since the concentration of ATP is very low in muscle, it is possible to deplete it rapidly in highly intense exercise. The depletion rate of ATP during intense activity would be much greater if it were not for creatine phosphate (CP) serving as a reservoir of phosphate units. The breakdown CP sustains ATP concentrations by the donation of the phosphate group from CP to ADP during the simultaneous breakdown of ATP. The breakdown of CP serves to sustain ATP levels in the muscle until the CP reservoir is itself depleted. When the reservoir is depleted, ATP concentration decreases precipitously, and so does the power output of the activity. In essence, the runner in a 200-meter run cannot complete the event at 40-meter sprint velocities, because of rapidly declining ATP concentrations. Muscle cells, in effect, run out of energy (ready ATP supply) and sprint velocity necessarily falls off. Without the presence of the next anaerobic metabolic pathway a 200-meter run could not be completed with much intensity of effort at all, and neither could anaerobic activities of longer duration such as the 400-meter run.

Two hundred meter sprints and races of longer distances can be completed in a very intense fashion due to the fact that our muscles have the capability to break down glucose to produce ATP in intense activity. The breakdown of glucose is termed glycolysis. During intense activity, longer than 10 to 15 seconds, exercising muscles rely more and more on glycolysis to pick up where the phosphagen system left off. This has very important implications, because without glucose breakdown during intense activity we would have to severely curtail our running velocity before we finished our 200-meter sprint. In effect, our range of anaerobic activities would be limited to those activities that could be completed with a very high intensity of effort before our res- ervoir of creatine phosphate ran out, which is only a few seconds. We would not be able to engage in the speed activities (intense activities that are more enduring than the power activities, but of much shorter duration than the endurance activities). Fortunately, the glycolytic pathway provides an adequate backup.

According to the concept of power versus capacity, glycolysis, while capable of supplying ATP very rapidly, is less powerful than the phosphagen system. One reason for this is that glycolysis is a far more complicated metabolic pathway. It involves the use of eleven enzymes, whereas the phosphagen system needs only two to produce ATP.

Remember that when power is low, capacity is high. This means that the capacity of glycolysis to produce ATP is much greater than the phosphagen system. The reason for this is that there is a lot more energy reserve stored as glucose, so much so that its storage quantity is not a limiting factor for intense activity. This means that glycolysis will be limited or forced to cease during intense activity prior to glucose being depleted in the cell. Recall that the reason ATP production via creatine phosphate breakdown stopped was that creatine phosphate exists in very limited quantities in muscle. These concepts make glycolysis an ideal backup to the phosphagen system in producing ATP anaerobically, greatly increasing our range of anaerobic activities.

The cell's capacity for glycolysis is crucial beyond the initial 10 to 15 seconds of very intense activity and up to approximately 90 seconds. However, there is a limit to the ability of glycolysis to sustain ATP production in intense activity. This limitation is brought about by the end product of glycolysis during intense activi- ties, lactic acid. When glucose is metabolized in muscle during intense activity, lactic acid, formed in the last of 11 reactions, increases in concentration in the muscle and spills over in the blood circulating through the muscle. Since this is an acid buildup, the pH of the cell significantly decreases to the point at which muscle contraction begins to be compromised due to at least two reasons. First, the buildup of acid in the muscle cell causes any further chemical breakdown of glucose to be hampered by decreasing the activity of the enzymes responsible for glucose breakdown. Second, as the watery medium of the muscle cell (the sarcoplasm) becomes more acidic, the ability of the muscle to continue to contract forcibly is reduced. The net result of this is that exercise intensity (i.e., running speed) must be reduced.

Lactic acid is a fatiguing substance and in this respect its buildup is detrimental. However, the ability of the cell to form lactic acid early in intense activity is actually what provides the cell with the capability to continue to make ATP rapidly. Therefore, lactic acid can be seen as necessary initially and detrimental later in intense activity.

Aerobic Production of ATP

When exercise is at an intensity level that can be maintained continuously for long periods of time, ATP is produced in muscles through cellular respiration, a process that uses oxygen. In terms of power versus capacity, the aerobic production of ATP has by far the least power. It is not capable of providing ATP rapidly. In turn, the capacity of this system far exceeds the anaerobic systems. Glycolysis releases only approximately 5% of the energy in the glucose molecule when its final product is lactic acid. When the exercise intensity is lower, the rest of this energy is liberated by cellular processes that are located in the mitochondria. Glucose breakdown continues in the mitochondria during activity that can be extended for long periods of time.

The processes of cellular respiration are very complex, involving the integration of cellular aerobic metabolism with several organ systems designed to coordinate fuel (energy nutrient) and oxygen delivery to the working muscles. Cellular respiration involves five separate metabolic pathways in the breakdown of the two main energy nutrients (triglyceride and glucose) used during steady-state (endurance) exercise.

The breakdown of triglycerides is termed lipolysis, a process that liberates fatty acids from the triglyceride molecule. This takes place primarily in adipose tissue. The fatty acids are released to the blood and transported to muscle cells where they are metabolized. The breakdown of fatty acids is termed beta-oxidation. In this process acctyl CoA is formed. Other pathways involved in the aerobic production of ATP are the Krebs cycle and the electron transport chain.

Beta oxidation and glycolysis are coordinated in that both funnel their end products to the respiratory mechanisms inside the mitochondria. Beta-oxidation ends in the formation of acetyl-CoA. Unlike the form of glycolysis that runs during intense activity, ending in lactic acid buildup, the form of glycolysis that proceeds during endurance activity ends in the formation of pyruvate. Pyruvate is placed into the mitochondria where it is also converted to acetyl-CoA. Therefore, acetyl-CoA is referred to as the common degradation product, because it is derived from both carbohydrate and fat catabolism. In the aerobic production of ATP during endurance-types of activities, both glucose and fats are metabolized simultaneously with common end prod- ucts entering cellular respiration in the mitochondria.

The aerobic production of ATP is far more complicated, because these reactions involve many separate metabolic pathways each with many enzyme steps that are located in different parts of the cell and the body. For instance, fatty acids are mobilized from fat cells during lipolysis and are catalyzed via beta oxidation in muscle during exercise. Muscle stores of triglycerides are also used. Recall that both anaerobic pathways were located in the sarcoplasm of the muscle fiber and had relatively few steps. This allowed ATP to be produced very rapidly for quick muscular activity. Thus, power was increased at the expense of capacity. In the aerobic system this is turned around, with the advantage now toward capacity. Also, now that fat is being utilized as a fuel substrate, the energy source is almost unlimited. This great increase in capacity, however, comes at the expense of decreases in power.

In many ways the Krebs cycle can be considered the beginning of the aerobic system, since it is the point of entry for all metabolic intermediate compounds that serve as fuel substrate to be completely broken down in cellular respiration. Starting in the Krebs cycle these compounds are further broken down to form additional energy-rich carrier molecules—nicotinamide adenine dinucleotide (NADH) and flavin adenine dinucleotide (FADH). These high-energy carrier molecules funnel hydrogen ions to the inner mitochondrial wall where the electron transport chain makes large quantities of ATP molecules in a process called oxidative phosphorylation (as opposed to substrate level phosphorylation when ATP was formed during glycolysis).

The Krebs cycle is also significant because it is the process whereby carbon dioxide is produced. The aerobic system is aptly named since a regular supply of oxygen is needed in the mitochondria to serve as a final reposi- tory for the hydrogen atoms that are stripped off of the energy nutrients during metabolism. With enough oxygen, NADH, and FADH present, oxygen serves as the final acceptor of hydrogen atoms as these atoms are passed along a series of intermediate acceptors. Throughout this process

ATP is generated, and metabolic water is produced. This process, therefore, utilizes the oxygen that we breathe in and deliver to the working muscles. In this process oxygen is said to be consumed.

The Cardiorespiratory System

Major organ systems must provide an adequate supply of oxygen to meet the demand contracting muscles have for oxygen during endurance exercise. The organ system that absorbs oxygen from the atmosphere and into blood is the pulmonary system. The cardiovascular system then delivers oxygen carried by the blood to the working muscles and all other organ systems. The heart and lungs are controlled to precisely match the increased metabolic demand for oxygen that occurs with exercise. These systems work as a unit to maintain oxygen and carbon dioxide homeostasis in the body.

The integration of the pulmonary and cardiovascular systems in the delivery, extraction, and utilization of oxygen can be depicted by an equation that expresses the relationship between three important variables: Oxygen consumption, cardiac output, and the arteriovenous oxygen difference. The blood delivered depends on the size of the cardiac output (the volume of blood circulated per minute). The amount of oxygen extracted depends in large part by the ability of the muscles to absorb and utilize oxygen. The three variables are shown in the equation below.

Oxygen Consumption = Cardiac Output		Arteriovenous Oxygen Difference
(Utilization) = (Amount Delivered)	×	(Amount Extracted)
Central Factor (Heart)		Peripheral Factor (Tissues)

There is an immediate need to meet the increased demand for oxygen with an adequate supply during endurance exercise. Heart rate and strength of cardiac contractions increase so that the cardiac output closely matches any level of oxygen consumption. The increased strength of cardiac contractions produces a greater cardiac stroke volume. Cardiac output is the product of heart rate and stroke volume. These factors result in an increase in the delivery of blood to the working muscles, and constitute the central factor (pertaining to the heart itself) for the increase in oxygen consumption that occurs with exercise. The increased delivery of blood is accomplished not only by an increase in blood flow (cardiac output), but by the massive redistribution of blood away from areas that do not participate in producing movement (the gastrointestinal tract, bone, skin) and toward the working muscles (where the greatest demand is). The increase in cardiac output, heart rate, and oxygen consumption during endurance activities is proportional to exercise intensity. For instance, both car- diac output and oxygen consumption increase in a step-by-step fashion as walking or running rate increases. However, during weightlifting, a resistance exercise that requires the anaerobic production of ATP, oxygen consumption is much lower for a given level of heart rate.

Second, as exercise intensity increases more oxygen is extracted from the blood as the blood passes through the capillaries of the working muscles. This can be measured as a larger difference between the oxygen content of the arteries feeding the muscles and oxygen content of the veins leaving the muscles. This greater difference in the oxygen content of arteries versus veins constitutes the peripheral (away from the heart) factor for the increase in oxygen consumption that occurs with exercise.

Third, the increase in oxygen consumption with exercise results from an increase in pulmonary ventilation. Pulmonary ventilation is the bulk flow of air into and out of the lungs. Upon the initiation of exercise the rate and depth of breathing increase, which results in an increase in pulmonary ventilation. As the exercise intensity during endurance activity increases, more air is passed in and out of the lungs. The increased rate at which the lungs are ventilated allows more oxygen to be delivered to the working muscles.

Thermoregulation

Mammals are classified as homeothermic, meaning that regardless of the state of the external environment, they must maintain internal body temperatures within narrow limits for survival. This is often quite challenging when faced with extremes of temperatures. One of the functions of the cardiovascular system is to remove heat from the body. This function is especially important during aerobic exercise, because of the large amount of heat produced and subsequently trapped in the body.

Part of the energy liberated during aerobic exercise is used to perform useful work. However, this portion of the energy expenditure is relative small (only about 20%–30%). This means that the remaining part of the energy produced is stored as heat and must be eliminated to maintain core temperature within reasonable levels. If this is not done adequately, the result may be some form of heat illness or possibly even death.

When aerobic exercise is performed in environmental conditions that are favorable (low to moderate air temperature and relative humidity), the body's ability to thermoregulate is sufficient to keep core temperature increases to a minimum. The increase in core temperature is linked to exercise intensity (as the percentage of maximal oxygen consumption). Exercise at 50% maximal oxygen consumption would mean a core tempera- ture increase of only 1 °C. This represents a successful thermoregulatory effort.

If environmental conditions are at the extremes of temperature, relative humidity, or both, thermoregulation is much harder to accomplish. The result of exercising in environmental extremes is an increased core temperature and a reduced work output. The reduced work output is a direct result of the extra burden placed on the cardiovascular system, which must not only supply oxygen to the working muscles to sustain the work output, but now it has an even more important role in delivering heat to the superficial regions of the body to dissipate the heat. This would have the direct effect of reducing maximal oxygen consumption and reducing exercise performance. In this case two areas of the body are competing for same cardiac output: the muscles to sustain the exercise intensity and the skin to dissipate the heat being carried by the blood. As the skin region receives more of the cardiac output, there is of necessity a reduction in endurance performance.

The ability to adequately dissipate the extra heat produced during aerobic exercise depends on the evaporative transfer of heat to the environment as water is vaporized from the respiratory passages and from the surface of the skin. Evaporation of water (sweat) off the skin is especially important since it represents the major way heat is removed from the body during exercise, except in hot, humid environments. Anything that retards this process will hinder exercise performance and carries a certain amount of risk to the exercising subject.

Evaporation is aided when the vapor pressure gradient from the skin surface to the air is large. This occurs when the relative humidity of the air is low. In this condition sweat easily evaporates to air that is relatively more dry than the skin. As water evaporates from the skin, heat is also transferred to the surroundings, and the body is cooled. Exercising in conditions of low relative humidity is, therefore, desirable. This problem is also independent of environmental temperatures since deaths have occurred in high humidity conditions even when temperatures have been moderate.

Inappropriate clothing greatly retards the evaporation of sweat from the skin. Different types of clothing are more effective in setting up a microenvironment around the skin than others, resulting in evaporation being retarded even when the outside environmental conditions are favorable. Certain types of athletic wear are specifically designed to provide a vapor barrier that completely stops the evaporative cooling process.

One of the most important things that can be done when exercising in a hot environment is to drink enough water. Studies have shown that water replacement is very effective in keeping the increase in core temperature seen with aerobic exercise to a minimum. When water balance (water intake that matched water loss) is maintained core body temperature increases are minimal.

Exercise Immunology

Exercise immunology is a dynamic developing sub-discipline of sports medicine. Although the knowledge about the diverse relationship between exercise and the immune system is profound, the complexity of immunity and its bidirectional interactions with other physiological systems continuously represents an enormous challenge.

Effects of Exercise on Infection Risk

Since early reports on a higher incidence of infections of the upper respiratory tract (URTI) in endurance athletes after periods of intensified training and competitions and the development of the open window theory, immunology research focused primarily on the acute and chronic effects of different types of exercise on immune system parameters and the identification of potential key risk factors. During the last years, there is increasing evidence, which challenges this theory. On the other hand, it is generally accepted that regular and moderate physical exercise improves the hosts immunocompetence and protects against infectious diseases. Therefore a distinction is made between the athlete's population and a public health perspective.

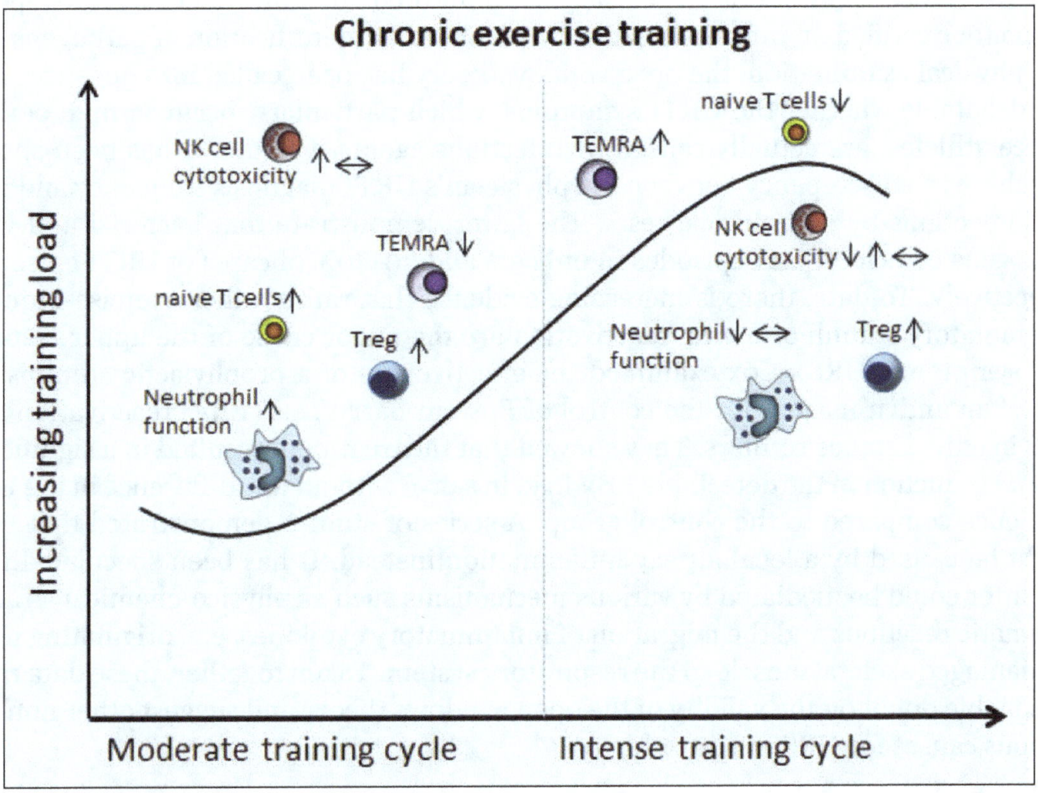

The most frequent illnesses in athletes are URTI and these infections are more likely to occur during intense training cycles and after tapering or after competitions than having seasonal patterns. There are early reports showing a 2-6-fold increase in the reported symptoms of URTI for several weeks after running a marathon and an association with the individual running time. Most of the evidence initially originated from studies, which involved running disciplines, but a series of data has confirmed the association between heavy exercise and URTI in other sports. Subsequently, much effort has been spent to the identification of potential mechanisms and risk factors for the increased URTI susceptibility in athletes.

However, it is challenging to interpret the clinical impact of changes in single immune system parameters because the immune system as a whole developed great redundancy. Nevertheless, a number of studies have shown that an acute bout of exercise, depending on mode, intensity and duration, is associated with a transient change in numerous immune system parameters such as peripheral leukocyte numbers and function or saliva immunoglobulin concentration. A genetic basis for a higher susceptibility to URTI has been proposed by both exercise and non-exercise studies demonstrating that the regulation of several anti-inflammatory pro-inflammatory cytokines is characteristic for illness prone individuals. Findings from studies investigating mucosal immune system (MIS) integrity are more controversial, as some reported on associations between saliva Immunoglobulin A (sIgA) concentrations and URTI incidence while others did not.

However, since many studies from the past monitored URTI incidence by self-reports but neither verified an infectious cause by a laboratory identification of pathogens nor by a physical examination, the open window theory has been called into question. It is still debatable whether the URTI symptoms, which particularly occur in high performance athletes, are actually caused by infectious agents. Further, it has been shown that there is a discrepancy between the physician's URTI diagnosis frequency and verified infections by pathological tests. The latter demonstrate that bacterial and viral pathogens coincide URTI episodes in only 5% and 30-40% of cases of URTI episodes, respectively. To date, there is increasing evidence that rather other exercise-induced inflammatory stimuli or a viral reactivation are the major cause of the upper respiratory symptoms (URS). Cox examined the effectiveness of a prophylactic administration of an antiviral agent for the control of Epstein Barr Virus (EBV) reactivation and URS in elite distance runners. They showed that the treatment resulted in a significant (-82%) reduction in the detectable EBV load in saliva without any difference in the URS incidence compared to the control group. A series of studies demonstrated that URS might be caused by a local airway inflammation instead. It has been speculated that the latter could be mediated by various mechanisms such as physico-chemical strains, asthmatic reactions and the migration of inflammatory cytokines, e.g. originating from the damaged skeletal muscle to the respiratory system. Taken together, these data raise reasonable doubt on the validity of the open windows theory and suggest other non-infectious causes for URS in elite athletes.

Apart from that, even if opportunistic infections are causative for URS in athletes, it is believed that additional/or other internal and external factors which precede or parallel episodes of intensified training or competition, such as mental stress and anxiety, sleep disruption, traveling, nutritional deficiencies, and exposure to climatic changes etc. likely play a key role in the impaired immune competence. Additionally, endurance competitions per se increase the risk of acquiring novel infections due to the exposure to human crowds. Apart from the detrimental effects of exhaustive exercise periods, there is limited evidence that master athletes are predisposed to have rather a more efficacious immune defense as they suffer from fewer URTI episodes, which allows them to realize higher training volumes and thereby to compete more successfully. It is speculated that beside genetic factors this population is characterized by behavioral factors such as a more effective hygiene routine, diet, sleep and stress management. Nevertheless, illness frequencies in athletic populations do not appear to be higher than in the general population but they do not show such a typical relationship of symptom episodes to seasonal patterns.

Beside from athletic populations and competitive sports, regular exercise training is a major protective factor as it ameliorates immune function, whereas a sedentary life-style depresses immunity. Both experimental and epidemiological research studies indicate a negative relationship between activity level and both, URTI incidence and the severity of URTI symptoms. In a 12-month observational study Matthews et al. evaluated the activity level of 547 healthy adults (age 20-70 years). After adjustment for a number of potential confounders including age, education, psychosocial measures and dietary factors, they showed that moderate levels of physical activity reduce the risk of URTI about 20%. Nonetheless, due to methodological limitations in the majority of research studies, it is impossible to determine the effectiveness of exercise in altering the occurrence, severity, or duration of URS to date.

Effects of Acute Exercise on Leukocyte Numbers and Function

Acute bouts of exercise are well-known to modulate the innate as well as adaptive immune response by affecting immune cell numbers and functions. Basically, the innate immune response represents the first line of defense against harmful pathogens and consists of cellular components such as granulocytes, macrophages, natural killer cells (NK), dendritic cells (DC) as well as soluble factors such as complement proteins among others. As an essential part of the innate immune response, granulocyte neutrophils represent a type of granula-secreting phagocytes that migrate to the inflamed tissue as first-responders to inflammatory cells. Acute exercise induces a first rapid neutrophilia, followed by a second delayed rise of blood neutrophil count a few hours later, depending on the duration and intensity of exercise. Novel findings let assume that the priming of neutrophils may be implicated in skeletal muscle inflammation after high-intensity exercise. On a functional level, unstimulated neutrophils respond to acute exercise stress with increased degranulation, oxidative burst and phagocytosis.

Additionally, after endurance exercise, the concentration of some complement proteins, such as C5a, is increased in the peripheral blood, promoting the chemotaxis of neutrophils. Monocytes are the largest type of blood leukocytes that can differentiate into macrophages or DCs after migration into damaged tissues and serve phagocytosis, antigen-presentation and cytokine production. With regard to monocytes, acute exercise induces a transient monocytosis of approximately two hours which is most likely due to a shift of monocytes from the marginalized to the circulating pool. Preferentially, acute exercise stimulates the mobilization of the proinflammatory CD14+/CD16+ monocyte subtype relative to classical CD14+/CD16- monocytes. To date, there is still a lack of studies investigating the exercise-induced mobilization of DCs, which act in the initiation of immune response by antigen presentation.

Interestingly, a recent study demonstrated a near fourfold increase of the number of monocyte-derived DCs (mo-DCs) after dynamic running exercise until volitional exhaustion without comprise of functional parameters. Since DCs are characterized by their unique ability to cross-present viral and tumor antigens, repetitive bouts of acute exercise might promote beneficial effects for health. NK cells are a minor subpopulation of lymphocytes which exhibit cytotoxicity and secrete cytokines promoting defense mechanisms against tumor- and virus-infected cells. Similarly to other blood leukocytes, NK-cells show a rapid mobilization in response to an acute bout of exercise. Preferentially, the cytotoxic CD56dim NK cell subset rather than the INF-Y the cytotoxic CD56dim NK cell subset rather than the INF-Y the cytotoxic CD56dim NK cell subset rather than the INFproducing CD56bright subtype appears to be mobilized by exercise. Moreover, functional changes in NK cell cytotoxicity depend on the intensity and duration of exercise. While short bouts of low- to moderate intensity exercise induce an increase, NK cell cytotoxicity expressed on a per cell basis can be reduced for hours after exhausting and prolonged exercise, probably favoring an increased susceptibility to infectious diseases.

Contrary to the innate immune response, the adaptive immunity is characterized by antigenic specificity and immunological memory and is composed of two main types of lymphocytes termed T cells and B cells. T cells are derived from the bone marrow and migrate to the thymus, where MHC-receptors are formed on their surface, allowing them to identify specifically foreign antigens. Furthermore, the differentiation process includes the maturation into diverse subpopulations such as CD4+ T-helper, CD8+ cytotoxic and regulatory T cells (Treg). B cells are the carriers of the humoral immune response and are the only cells capable of producing antibodies after differentiation into plasma cells. Acute exercise results in transient biphasic changes in the numbers of circulating lymphocytes marked by lymphocytosis during and immediately after exercise, while numbers of cells sinking below basal levels during the early recovery period.

Studies indicate that the initial increase of lymphocytes may be the result of mobilization from the marginal pool, the spleen as well as other lymphoid tissues, while the exercise-induced lymphopenia in the post-exercise period seems to be due to redistribution in lymphoid- and non-lymphoid organs and apoptosis. Particularly, exercise-induced mobilization of T cells seems to be affected by differentiation stage. Accordingly, highly differentiated T cells show a more frequent mobilization response to acute exercise compared to low differentiated T cells. Unlike T cells, B cell mobilization does not seem to be triggered by effector status. In response to acute exercise, the immature B cell subpopulation displays the largest increase, followed by memory B cells and naïve B cells.

However, recent studies reveal that the behavior of the exercise-induced mobilization of differentiated T cells is highly dependent on exercise intensity, training status, and individual predispositions such as CMV serostatus and age. Thus, high-intensity loads induce greater apoptosis in highly differentiated T cells than moderate intensity exercise. Moreover, high physical fitness individuals show a greater decrease of mobilized highly differentiated effector memory T cells (mTeff) in the early post-exercise period, possibly indicating more efficient clearance mechanisms. Independently of exercise intensity CMV-seronegative athletes mobilize more low- and medium differentiated T cells than CMV-seropositive. Further, the amount of CD34+ hematopoietic progenitor cells and angiogenic T cells (TANG) is inversely correlated with age and older adults display attenuated exercise-induced mobilization of these cell t ypes.

To date, only a limited number of studies are available investigating the effects of acute exercise on Treg cells. Tregs are a specialized subgroup of T cells that modulate the activation of the immune system by suppressing the activation and proliferation of effector T-cells as well as maintaining tolerance to self-antigens. Novel studies demonstrated that Treg cells are mobilized in response to high-intensity exercise stress. In this context, a higher level of physical fitness appears to promote a stronger mobilization. On the one hand, Treg mobilization amplifies exercise-induced immunosuppression, but on the other hand, it may also have immune regulatory effects.

Kinesiology

Kinesiology encompasses holistic health disciplines which use the gentle art of muscle monitoring to access information about a person's well being. Originating in the 1970's, it combines Western techniques and Eastern wisdom to promote physical, emotional,mental and spiritual health. Kinesiology identifies the elements which inhibit the body's natural internal energies and accessing the life enhancing potential within the individual".

Kinesiology is a non-invasive energetic healing science. Initial research began in the 1960's when Dr. George Goodheart DC, discovered that muscle testing could be used to gather information from the body. This system was called 'Applied Kinesiology' and saw many chiropractors embracing Chinese medicine techniques of acupressure and meridian systems.

Kinesiology, which is a combination of ancient, eastern science and western muscle monitoring, balances the body on many levels. Its effective results come from the way it works with the body's innate healing intelligence to restore balance and health to neurological and physiological function. Through this modality, profound changes may be experienced emotionally, mentally and physically, thereby increasing a person's health and wellbeing. When our system is functioning well, we feel well.

Professional Kinesiology practitioners undertake years of training to be able to access the movement of energy - or what the Chinese call 'Chi' - throughout the body. The analogy of a bio-computer illustrates in a simple manner how this works.

Blocks or stresses prevent smooth energetic transmission, thus affecting functioning of our biosystems, resulting in changes in energy. Muscle monitoring involves challenging the biofeedback mechanism present in all muscles to reveal imbalances within the body. The 'read out', or findings, may present as physical pain, mental discomfort and the many expressions of disease. These can include allergies, depression, postural problems, poor performance levels, learning and relationship difficulties, digestive and nervous disorders - whatever the presenting problem, the system is saying it is malfunctioning.

The real goal of any Kinesiology 'balance' is to identify the bottomline cause of any imbalance and then resolve it. It may be nutritional, emotional, structural, psychological, energetic or even spiritual - something as simple as an 'attitude', or a forgotten memory.

Muscle monitoring gives instant access to holistic information held by the core operating unit of the entire body-mind system - the subconscious. This normally inaccessible neural substrate holds all our memories, information about physical, emotional, mental and energetic states, and also determines our muscle tension. Accessing the bio-system, allows the Kinesiologist to quickly determine the specific strategy to best reinstate to the body's balance.

At subtle levels, the person is already aware of what is needed to facilitate healing. What kinesiology is able to do, in a therapeutic sense, is to access that information in order to assist the natural healing process.

Adaptation and Physiologic Responses to Exercise

When challenged with any physical task, the human body responds through a series of integrated changes in function that involve most, if not all, of its physiologic systems. Movement requires activation and control of the musculoskeletal system; the cardiovascular and respiratory systems provide the ability to sustain this movement over extended periods. When the body engages in exercise training several times a week or more frequently, each of these physiologic systems undergoes specific adaptations that increase the body's efficiency and capacity. The magnitude of these changes depends largely on the intensity and duration of the training sessions, the force or load used in training, and the body's initial level of fitness. Removal of the training stimulus, however, will result in loss of the efficiency and capacity that was gained through these training-induced adaptations; this loss is a process called detraining.

Physiologic Responses to Episodes of Exercise

The body's physiologic responses to episodes of aerobic and resistance exercise occur in the musculoskeletal, cardiovascular, respiratory, endocrine, and immune systems. These responses have been studied in controlled laboratory settings, where exercise stress can be precisely regulated and physiologic responses carefully observed.

Cardiovascular and Respiratory Systems

The primary functions of the cardiovascular and respiratory systems are to provide the body with oxygen (O_2) and nutrients, to rid the body of carbon dioxide (CO_2) and metabolic waste products, to maintain body temperature and acid-base balance, and to transport hormones from the endocrine glands to their target organs. To be effective and efficient, the cardiovascular system should be able to respond to increased skeletal muscle activity. Low rates of work, such as walking at 4 kilometers per hour (2.5 miles per hour), place relatively small demands on the cardio- vascular and respiratory systems. However, as the rate of muscular work increases, these two systems will eventually reach their maximum capacities and will no longer be able to meet the body's demands.

Cardiovascular Responses to Exercise

The cardiovascular system, composed of the heart, blood vessels, and blood, responds predictably to the increased demands of exercise. With few exceptions, the cardiovascular response to exercise is directly proportional to the skeletal muscle oxygen demands for any given rate of work, and oxygen uptake ($\dot{V}O_2$) increases linearly with increasing rates of work.

Cardiac Output

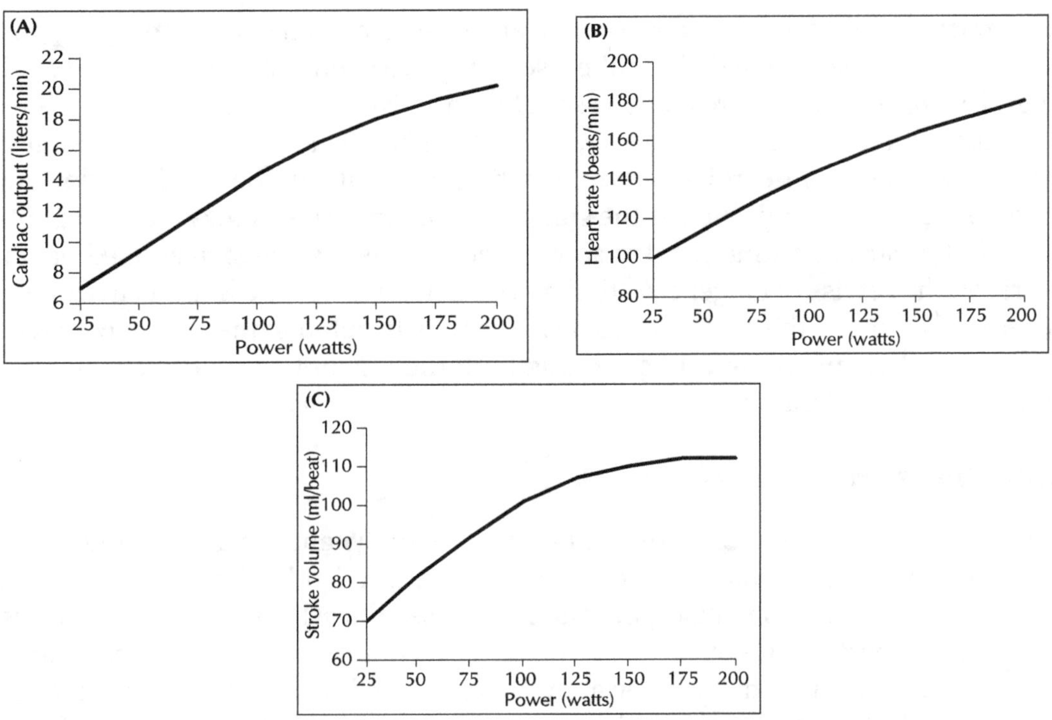

Changes in (A) cardiac output, (B) heart rate and (C) stroke volume with increasing rates of work on the cycle ergometer.

Cardiac output ($\dot{Q}$) is the total volume of blood pumped by the left ventricle of the heart per minute. It is the product of heart rate (HR, number of beats per minute) and stroke volume (SV, volume of blood pumped per beat). The arterial-mixed venous oxygen($A-\overline{v}O_2$) difference is the difference between the oxy-gen content of the arterial and mixed venous blood. A person's maximum oxygen uptake ($\dot{V}O_2$ max) is a function of cardiac output ($\dot{Q}$) multiplied by the $A-\overline{v}O_2$ difference. Cardiac output thus plays an important role in meeting the oxygen demands for work. As the rate of work increases, the cardiac output increases in a nearly linear manner to meet the increasing oxygen demand, but only up to the point where it reaches its maximal capacity ($\dot{Q}$max).

To visualize how cardiac output, heart rate, and stroke volume change with increasing rates of work, consider a person exercising on a cycle ergometer, starting at 50 watts and increasing 50 watts every 2 minutes up to a maximal rate of work. In this scenario, cardiac output and heart rate increase over the entire range of work, whereas stroke volume only increases up to approximately 40 to 60 present of the person's maximal oxygen uptake($\dot{V}O_2$ max), after which it reaches a plateau. Recent studies have suggested that stroke volume in highly trained persons can continue to increase up to near maximal rates of work.

Blood Flow

The pattern of blood flow changes dramatically when a person goes from resting to exercising. At rest, the skin and skeletal muscles receive about 20 percent of the cardiac output. During exercise, more blood is sent to the active skeletal muscles, and, as body temperature increases, more blood is sent to the skin. This process is accomplished both by the increase in cardiac output and by the redistribution of blood flow away from areas of low demand, such as the splanchnic organs. This process allows about 80 percent of the cardiac output to go to active skeletal muscles and skin at maximal rates of work. With exercise of longer duration, particularly in a hot and humid environment, progressively more of the cardiac output will be redistributed to the skin to counter the increasing body temperature, thus limiting both the amount going to skeletal muscle and the exercise endurance.

Blood Pressure

Mean arterial blood pressure increases in response to dynamic exercise, largely owing to an increase in systolic blood pressure, because diastolic blood pressure remains at near-resting levels. Systolic blood pressure increases linearly with increasing rates of work, reaching peak values of between 200 and 240 millimeters of mercury in normotensive persons. Because mean arterial pressure is equal to cardiac output times total peripheral resistance, the observed increase in mean arterial pressure results from an increase in cardiac output that outweighs a concomitant decrease in total peripheral resistance. This increase in mean arterial pressure is a normal and desirable response, the result of a resetting of the arterial bar reflex to a higher pressure. Without such a resetting, the body would experience severe arterial hypotension during intense activity. Hypertensive patients typically reach much higher systolic blood pressures for a given rate of work, and they can also experience increases in diastolic blood pressure. Thus, mean arterial pressure is generally much higher in these patients, likely owing to a lesser reduction in total peripheral resistance.

For the first 2 to 3 hours following exercise, blood pressure drops below preexercise resting levels, a phenomenon referred to as post exercise hypotension. The specific mechanisms underlying this response have not been established. The acute changes in blood pressure after an episode of exercise may be an important aspect of the role of physical activity in helping control blood pressure in hypertensive patients.

Oxygen Extraction

The $A-\bar{v}O_2$ difference increases with increasing rates of work and results from increased oxygen extraction from arterial blood as it passes through exercising muscle. At rest, the $A-\bar{v}O_2$ differ ence is approximately 4 to 5 ml of O_2 for every 100 ml of blood (ml/100 ml); as the rate of work approaches maximal levels, the $A-\bar{v}O_2$ difference reaches 15 to 16 ml/100 ml of blood.

Coronary Circulation

The coronary arteries supply the myocardium with blood and nutrients. The right and left coronary arteries curve around the external surface of the heart, then branch and penetrate the myocardial muscle bed, dividing and subdividing like branches of a tree to form a dense vascular and capillary network to supply each myocardial muscle fiber. Generally one capillary supplies each myocardial fiber in adult humans and animals; however, evidence suggests that the capillary density of the ventricular myocardium can be increased by endurance exercise training.

At rest and during exercise, myocardial oxygen demand and coronary blood flow are closely linked. This coupling is necessary because the myocardium depends almost completely on aerobic metabolism and therefore requires a constant oxygen supply. Even at rest, the myocardium's oxygen use is high relative to the blood flow. About 70 to 80 percent of the oxygen is extracted from each unit of blood crossing the myocardial capillaries; by comparison, only about 25 percent is extracted from each unit crossing skeletal muscle at rest. In the healthy heart, a linear relationship exists between myocardial oxy- gen demands, consumption, and coronary blood flow, and adjustments are made on a beat-to-beat basis. The three major determinants of myocardial oxygen consumption are heart rate, myocardial contractility, and wall stress. Acute increases in arterial pressure increase left ventricular pressure and wall stress. As a result, the rate of myocardial metabolism increases, necessitating an increased coronary blood flow. A very high correlation exists between both myocardial oxygen consumption and coronary blood flow and the product of heart rate and systolic blood pressure (SBP). This so called double product (HR • SBP) is generally used to estimate myocardial oxygen and coronary blood flow requirements. During vigorous exercise, all three major determinants of myocardial oxygen requirements increase above their resting levels.

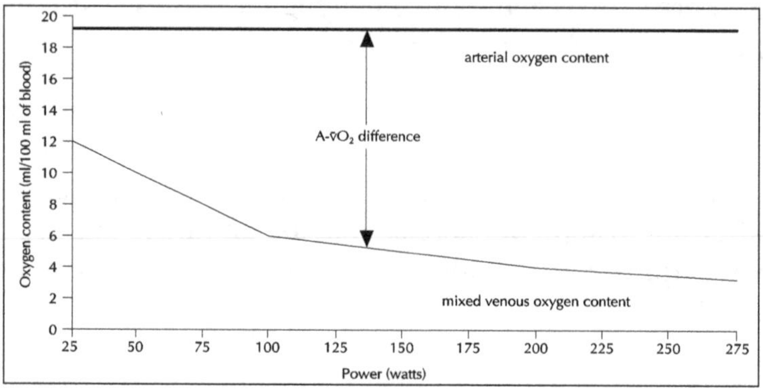

Changes in arterial and mixed venous oxygen content with increasing rates of work on the cycle ergometer.

The increase in coronary blood flow during exercise results from an increase in perfusion pressure of the coronary artery and from coronary vasodilation. Most important, an increase in sympathetic nervous system stimulation leads to an increase in circulating catecholamines. This response triggers metabolic processes that increase both perfusion pressure of the coronary artery and coronary vasodilation to meet the increased need for blood flow required by the increase in myocardial oxygen use.

Respiratory Responses to Exercise

The respiratory system also responds when challenged with the stress of exercise. Pulmonary ventilation increases almost immediately, largely through stimulation of the respiratory centers in the brain stem from the motor cortex and through feedback from the proprioceptors in the muscles and joints of the active limbs. During prolonged exercise, or at higher rates of work, increases in CO_2 production, hydrogen ions (H^+), and body and blood temperatures stimulate further increases in pulmonary ventilation. At low work intensities, the increase in ventilation is mostly the result of increases in tidal volume. At higher intensities, the respiratory rate also increases. In normal-sized, untrained adults, pulmonary ventilation rates can vary from about 10 liters per minute at rest to more than 100 liters per minute at maximal rates of work; in large, highly trained male athletes, pulmonary ventilation rates can reach more than 200 liters per minute at maximal rates of work.

Resistance Exercise

The cardiovascular and respiratory responses to episodes of resistance exercise are mostly similar to those associated with endurance exercise. One no- table exception is the exaggerated blood pressure response that occurs during resistance exercise. Part of this response can be explained by the fact that resistance exercise usually involves muscle mass that develops considerable force. Such high, isolated force leads to compression of the smaller arteries and results in substantial increases in total peripheral resistance. Although high-intensity resistance training poses a potential risk to hypertensive patients and to those with cardiovascular dis- ease, research data suggest that the risk is relatively low and that hypertensive persons may benefit from resistance training.

Skeletal Muscle

The primary purpose of the musculoskeletal system is to define and move the body. To provide efficient and effective force, muscle adapts to demands. In response to demand, it changes its ability to extract oxygen, choose energy sources, and rid itself of waste products. The body contains three types of muscle tissue: Skeletal (voluntary) muscle, cardiac muscle or myocardium, and smooth (autonomic) muscle.

Skeletal muscle is composed of two basic types of muscle fibers distinguished by their speed of contraction—slow-twitch and fast-twitch—a characteristic that is largely dictated by different forms of the enzyme myosin adenosinetriphosphatase (ATPase). Slow-twitch fibers, which have relatively slow contractile speed, have high oxidative capacity and fatigue resistance, low glycolytic capacity, relatively high blood flow capacity, high capillary density, and high mitochondrial content. Fast-twitch muscle fibers have fast contractile speed and are classified into two subtypes, fast-twitch type "a" ($FT_{a)}$ and fast-twitch type "b" (FT_b). FT_a fibers have moderately high oxidative capacity, are relatively fatigue resistant, and have high glycolytic capacity, relatively high blood flow capacity, high capillary density, and high mitochondrial content. FT_b fibers have low oxidative capacity, low fatigue resistance, high glycolytic capacity, and fast contractile speed. Further, they have relatively low blood flow capacity, capillary density, and mitochondrial content.

There is a direct relationship between predominant fiber type and performance in certain sports. For example, in most marathon runners, slow-twitch fibers account for up to or more than 90 percent of the total fibers in the leg muscles. On the other hand, the leg muscles in sprinters are often more than 80 percent composed of fast-twitch fibers. Although the issue is not totally resolved, muscle fiber type appears to be genetically determined; researchers have shown that several years of either high-intensity sprint training or high-intensity endurance training do not significantly alter the percentage of the two major types of fibers.

Skeletal Muscle Energy Metabolism

Metabolic processes are responsible for generating adenosine triphosphate (ATP), the body's energy source for all muscle action. ATP is generated by three basic energy systems: the ATP-phosphocreatine (ATP-PCr) system, the glycolytic system, and the oxidative system. Each system contributes to energy production in nearly every type of exercise. The relative contribution of each will depend on factors such as the intensity of work rate at the onset of exercise and the availability of oxygen in the muscle.

Energy Systems

The ATP-PCr system provides energy from the ATP stored in all of the body's cells. PCr, also found in all cells, is a high-energy phosphate molecule that stores energy. As ATP concentrations in the cell are reduced by the breakdown of ATP to adenosine diphosphate (ADP) to release energy for muscle contraction, PCr is broken down to release both energy and a phosphate to allow reconstitution of ATP from ADP. This process describes the primary energy system for short, high-intensity exercise, such as a 40- to 200-meter sprint; during such exercise, the system can produce energy at very high rates, and ATP and PCr stores, which are depleted in 10–20 seconds, will last just long enough to complete the exercise.

At high rates of work, the active muscle cell's oxygen demand exceeds its supply. The cell must then rely on the glycolytic energy system to produce ATP in the absence of oxygen (i.e., anaerobically). This system can only use glucose, available in the blood plasma and stored in both muscle and the liver as glycogen. The glycolytic energy system is the primary energy system for all-out bouts of exercise lasting from 30 seconds to 2 minutes, such as an 800-meter run. The major limitation of this energy system is that it produces lactate, which lowers the pH of both the muscle and blood. Once the pH drops below a value of 6.4 to 6.6, enzymes critical for producing energy are no longer able to function, and ATP production stops.

The oxidative energy system uses oxygen to produce ATP within the mitochondria, which are special cell organelles within muscle. This process cannot generate ATP at a high enough rate to sustain an all-out sprint, but it is highly effective at lower rates of work (e.g., long distance running). ATP can also be produced from fat and protein metabolism through the oxidative energy system. Typically, carbohydrate and fat provide most of the ATP; under most conditions, protein contributes only 5 to 10 percent at rest and during exercise.

Metabolic Rate

The rate at which the body uses energy is known as the metabolic rate. When measured while a person is at rest, the resulting value represents the lowest (i.e., basal) rate of energy expenditure necessary to maintain basic body functions. Resting metabolic rate is measured under highly controlled resting conditions following a 12-hour fast and a good night's sleep. To quantify the rate of energy expenditure during exercise, the metabolic rate at rest is defined as 1 metabolic equivalent (MET); a 4 MET activity thus represents an activity that requires four times the resting metabolic rate. The use of METs to quantify physical activity intensity is the basis of the absolute intensity scale.

Maximal Oxygen Uptake

During exercise, ($\dot{V}O_2$) increases in direct proportion to the rate of work. The point at which a person's $V^{\cdot}O_2$ is no longer able to increase is defined as the maximal oxygen uptake ($\dot{V}O_2$ max). A person's $\dot{V}O_2$ max is in part genetically determined; it can be increased through training until the point that the genetically possible maximum is reached. $\dot{V}O_2$ max is considered the best estimate of a person's cardio-respiratory fitness or aerobic power.

Lactate Threshold

Lactate is the primary by-product of the anaerobic glycolytic energy system. At lower exercise intensities, when the cardiorespiratory system can meet the oxygen demands of active muscles, blood lactate levels remain close to those observed at rest, because some lactate is used aerobically by muscle and is removed as fast as it enters the blood from the muscle. As the intensity of exercise is increased, however, the rate of lactate entry into the blood from muscle eventually exceeds its rate of removal from the blood, and blood lactate concentrations increase above resting levels. From this point on, lactate levels continue to increase as the rate of work increases, until the point of exhaustion. The point at which the concentration of lactate in the blood begins to increase above resting levels is referred to as the lactate threshold.

Lactate threshold is an important marker for endurance performance, because distance runners set their race pace at or slightly above the lactate threshold. Further, the lactate thresholds of highly trained endurance athletes occur at a much higher percentage of their $\dot{V}O_2$ max, and thus at higher relative workloads, than do the thresholds of untrained persons. This key difference is what allows endurance athletes to perform at a faster pace.

Hormonal Responses to Exercise

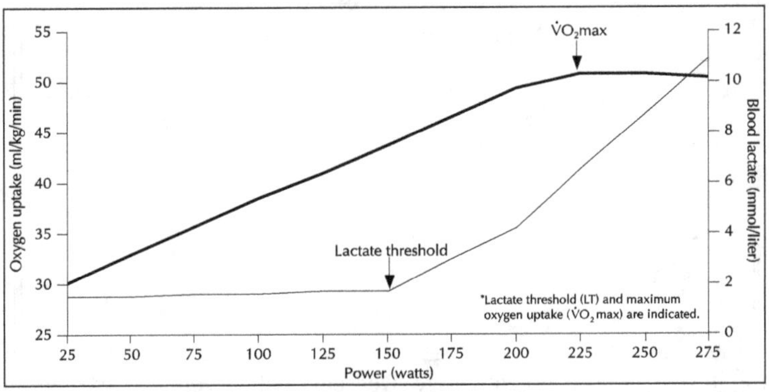

Changes in oxygen uptake and blood lactate concentrations with increasing rates of work on the cycle ergometer.

The endocrine system, like the nervous system, integrates physiologic responses and plays an important role in maintaining homeostatic conditions at rest and during exercise. This system controls the release of hormones from specialized glands through- out the body, and these hormones exert their actions on targeted organs and cells. In response to an episode of exercise, many hormones, such as catecholamines, are secreted at an increased rate, though insulin is secreted at a decreased rate.

Immune Responses to Exercise

The immune system is a complex adaptive system that provides surveillance against foreign proteins, viruses, and bacteria by using the unique functions of cells produced by the bone marrow and the thymus land. By interacting with neural and endocrine factors, the immune system influences the body's overall response to exercise. A growing body of literature indicates that the incidence of some infections may be influenced by the exercise history of the individual.

Moderate exercise has been shown to bolster the function of certain components of the human immune system—such as natural killer cells, circulating T- and B-lymphocytes, and cells of the monocyte-macrophage system—thereby possibly decreasing the incidence of some infections and perhaps of certain types of cancer.

Exercise of high intensity and long duration or exercise that involves excessive training may have adverse effects on immune function. In general, a high-intensity, single episode of exercise results in a marked decline in the functioning of all major cells of the immune system. In addition, over-training may reduce the response of T-lymphocytes to mutagenic stimulation, decrease antibody synthesis and plasma level of immunoglobins and complement, and impair macrophage phagocytosis. The reduced plasma glutamine levels that occur with high-intensity exercise or excessive training are postulated to contribute to these adverse effects on the immune system.

Neuroplasticity

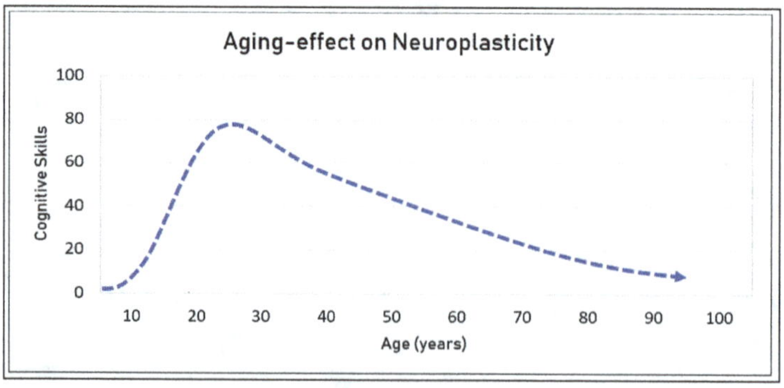

The gradual decline in brain cognition as we age. Decreases observed in reasoning, processing speed, working memory, and spatial orientation after mid-20s (Adapted from information in).

Neuroplasticity refers to the brains capacity to adapt and reorganise as we experience and learn different tasks. The scope of neuroplasticity is large and complex, with different events occurring at the molecular, synaptic, and muscular levels over short and long periods of time. However, neuroplasticity can be understood by strength and conditioning coaches through grasping basic information around the topic. To begin, we must learn about the role of gray matter and how it relates to the ability to acquire and retain motor skills.

Importance of Gray Matter

Our brain and spinal cord contain gray matter (GM) which is responsible for the motor control and sensory perception in our body. GM contains motor neurons which send action potentials down the axon and into our muscle cells, which results in movement. There tends to be a stronger signal and more refined neural pathway when there is high GM density in the brain. Studies indicate that humans tend to increase GM density during childhood, followed by a loss of GM density after puberty. It is suggested that as we mature, the volume of synaptic connections decreases and our ultimate GM density is determined.

An interesting study by Gogtay reports that following brain maturation an adolescent's GM density diminishes until young adulthood. However, this does not mean that we are unable to learn new motor patterns after puberty. Instead, it simply implies that the greatest "window of opportunity" for learning motor skills is before puberty, and that afterwards, motor skill pattern potential is limited due to the motor synapses closing.

Fast and Slow-stage Learning

Changes in motor skill neuroplasticity are often divided into a "fast-stage" (short-term) and "slow-stage" (long-term). During fast-stage learning, it is believed that the primary motor cortex in our brain recruits substantially more neurons for new motor tasks. This increase in brain activity can result in vast improvements being seen within a single training session. After improving at a motor skill, we transition to the slow-stage of learning where multiple training sessions and repetitive practice is needed to retain or improve that skill.

Unlike the fast-stage, the slow-stage of learning results in small improvements at a much slower pace. This is due to neuroplasticity's "use it or lose it" principle when it comes to motor skills. The brain's plasticity will either slowly strengthen or reduce a motor pathway based on repetitive action, or the lack-of. However, past repetitive practice of motor tasks could lead to a quicker re-adaptation if there was stoppage of that skill. This term is called "savings" and is why many athletes can still perform a skill such as shooting a basketball, even after years of not practicing.

One important thing to consider with fast-stage and slow-stage learning is that the acquisition of a skill is highly task-specific and relevant to the person. Generally, the learning curve of a motor skill will look the same when considering the specificity and difficulty of certain skills.

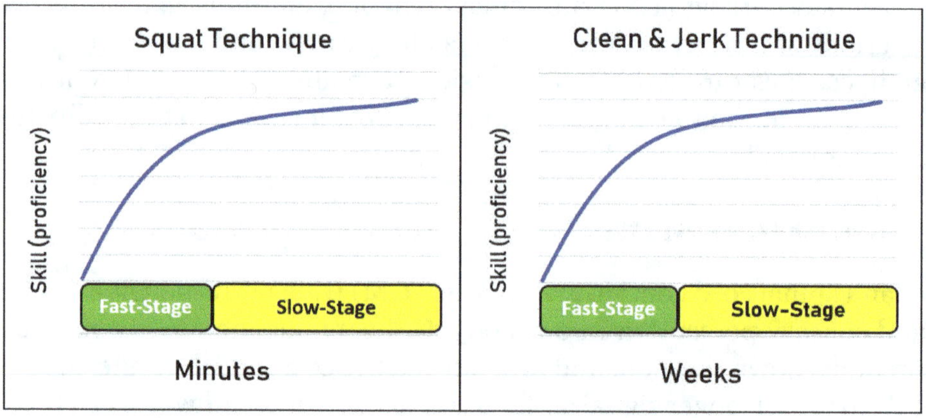

An example of the general learning curve for fast-stage and slow-stage learning of two different motor-skills (Adapted from).

Learning basic squat technique can be done within one training session with some athletes. The Clean & Jerk, however, can take weeks of practice in order to become proficient due to the coordination needed to perform the exercise at high speed. Of the two exercises, the Clean & Jerk is a much more difficult motor skill to learn, and whilst it would be unfair to compare the two exercises hand-in-hand, it does provide a clear example of movement complexity, skill acquisition, and the different times needed to learn certain movements.

Importance of Neuroplasticity for Sport

To proficiently perform athletic movements the brain must coordinate with the necessary muscle groups to produce the action. Whether the athlete is throwing a baseball, kicking a football, or even sprinting, these all require complex inter- and intra-muscular coordination which starts from the brains motor cortex. Therefore, repetitive practice is needed for a motor skill to be performed effectively, and thus engrained.

In most sporting competitions, athletes are at a disadvantage if they need to think before moving. Many people use the term "muscle memory" when they perform a skill automatically and without much thought. While incorrect, it does imply that a certain motor pathway is so well-developed that less brain activity and neuron organisation with the muscles is needed to perform a skill which before felt unaccustomed and alien. This is the reason why some skills tend to look or feel effortless after repetitive practice.

Due to neuroplasticity, every time a skill is performed our brain refines that motor pathway, regardless of whether it was performed correctly or incorrectly. For this reason, it is important to have coaches that promote correct technique, whether it be for the sport or in the weight room. If a bad movement pattern is performed repeatedly, the technique will require more practice and time to fix/refine. While neuroplasticity for sporting skills are achievable throughout our lives, research indicates that there is an opportune time to do so.

Neuroplasticity and Age

Plasticity in the brain appears to peak in prepubescent children, therefore, it may be the opportune time to capitalise on teaching correct technique/movement/skills. By introducing multiple motor skills to young children, they have the unique advantage of maximising and enhancing muscular strength and fundamental sporting skills which may not be available as adults. Training and exercise for young athletes should be specifically focused on improving motor control since their cognitive and motor capabilities are highly "plastic".

It has been suggested that integrative neuromuscular training (INT) be introduced during the childhood and adolescent time-period to influence the plasticity of the motor cortex which will carry into adulthood. INT are exercises that expose children to a variety of movement patterns and challenges that promote cognitive and physical development. By properly introducing and implementing INT, this will allow for the physical, mental, and social development which will positively affect athleticism as the child grows. If an athlete is not exposed to a certain motor skill prior to full motor cortex maturation, they are still capable of developing that skill, however, the benefit and potential is diminished.

Neuroplasticity with regards to motor skill is available during a human's entire lifespan, but is best retained during all developmental stages. Professionals that work in sport must implement training that teaches and reinforces good movement, regardless of age or training level. Much like the SAID (specific adaptations to imposed demands) principle in training, the motor cortex adapts in a similar way. Athletes should always be improving or refining their motor skills to maximise performance in competition.

Issues with Neuroplasticity

Measuring 'plasticity' in an athlete's brain is not worthwhile for strength and conditioning professionals for a few reasons. Examining neuroplasticity requires invasive and expensive equipment as imaging of gray matter and other regions of the brain require access to an MRI machine and medical professionals to operate it.

Also, most research surrounding neuroplasticity in motor skills is not done in athletes, rather individuals with movement disorders such as cerebral palsy and animals. Therefore, it may not meaningful to quantify brain 'plasticity' in athletes, when instead the focus should be on teaching and refining motor competency.

Evidence suggests that there are gender differences in the adolescent brain which can affect neuroplasticity. Research has reported that there is a higher ratio of GM to white matter in females and that they may also reach peak values of brain volume earlier than males. Similarly, it appears that the sex-hormones testosterone and estrogen also have gender-specific effects on the organisation of brain structure during puberty which may affect its development.

The concept of neuroplasticity does suggest repetitive practice of motor skills to strengthen and refine movement competency. Many have heard of the 10,000 hours rule proposed by Malcolm Gladwell, which suggests that this is the amount of time of deliberate practice needed to become phenomenal at a task. However, this is often taken out of context and drives people to over-train and eventually burn-out from exhaustion.

With neuroplasticity, there is a proposed concept of "offline training" which states that performance improvements of a skill can occur between training sessions with no further practice. It is believed that this is due to a phenomenon in which the brain consolidates a movement pattern at the end of every practice which progressively stabilises the skill. This results in an increase of accuracy, execution, and reaction of a motor skill due to rest.

"Offline" skill improvements can be affected by sleep, which ultimately demonstrates the importance of adequate rest/sleep. Therefore, mastery of a motor skill is likely to require a high-volume of deliberate training with sufficient rest between sessions and adequate sleep.

Motor Redundancy

Motor redundancy is a widely-used concept in kinesiology and motor control which states that for any task the human body can perform, there are effectively an unlimited number of ways the nervous system could achieve that task. This redundancy appears at multiple levels in the chain of motor execution.

Kinematic redundancy means that for a desired location of the endpoint (e.g. the hand or finger) there are many configurations of the joints that would produce the same endpoint location in space. Muscle redundancy means that the same net joint torque could be generated by many different relative contributions of individual muscles.

The concept of motor redundancy is explored in numerous studies usually with the goal of describing the relative contribution of a set of motor elements (e.g. muscles) in various human movements, and how these contributions can be predicted from a comprehensive theory. Two distinct (but not incompatible) theories have emerged for how the nervous system coordinates redundant elements: simplification and optimization. In the simplification theory, complex movements and muscle actions are constructed from simpler ones, often known as primitives or synergies, resulting in a simpler system for the brain to control. In optimization theory, motor actions arise from the minimization of control parameter, such as the energetic cost of movement or errors in movement performance.

Energy Balance

Energy balance is important for the human body to regulate the total amount of energy which it receives in the food eaten so that this will balance the total amount of energy which is expended. The sources of energy available to the body come from solid food plus fluids (such as milk, juices, or alcohol). There are several ways in which the body expends energy: most importantly (i) as the basal metabolic rate (BMR); (ii) in the processes of digestion and absorption of foodstuffs; and (iii) in physical activity. (i) The BMR is the total amount of energy expended when the body is apparently at rest: that is, it refers to the work of breathing, contraction of the heart, circulation of the blood, kidney function, and so on, including the metabolism of all the body's living cells. These are all essential functions and closely represent the minimal total metabolism of the body, though it may be further reduced during sleep. The BMR for an adult woman of average body size would be about 1400 kcal/day and for an average man about 1700 kcal/day. These amounts account for roughly 60–70% of the total daily energy expenditure.

There is considerable variability in BMR among individuals who are superficially similar, and since BMR accounts for a large portion of total energy metabolism, the extent of this variation can have important implications. For instance, two people who might appear to be physically similar in body weight and in body composition (with respect to the relative proportions of fat and lean) might differ in BMR by 300–400 kcal/day, meaning that one of them could eat food with an energy content of 300–400 kcal/day more than the other with the same end result for energy balance. In our present day Western lifestyle, this would impose a penalty on the biologically more efficient individual, whose BMR is comparatively low and who will therefore be somewhat unfairly constrained to a life of partial self-denial if obesity is to be avoided. The low BMR means that the total energy requirement of such a person will also be relatively low, compared with others with a similar pattern of physical activity, and will therefore be satisfied by a smaller total food intake — which may not be to that person's particular liking. The compensation for these people is a somewhat inadequate one in a privileged society; faced with a famine situation, they could expect to survive better and longer than those with average BMR. (ii) After a meal, the processes of *digestion and absorption* are initiated and continue for some hours. This involves an expenditure of some energy, equivalent to roughly 10% of the total calorie content of energy of the food and drink taken. The more food you eat, the more energy is used up in processing it. (iii) *Physical activity* obviously affects energy expenditure. Its influence on energy balance can go in either direction. With increased physical activity the extent of the greater energy expenditure will obviously depend on the intensity and duration of the exercise. If the energy expended is sufficiently large, this leads to a state of negative energy balance and part of the energy which would normally be supplied by the food will be obtained from the breakdown of energy stores (mostly from fat). The consequence is a reduction of body weight, and increased physical activity is indeed often prescribed as a treatment for obesity — albeit not always with marked success.

Energy Balance and Imbalance in Terms of a Biological System

Human physiology complies with the first law of thermodynamics, which states that energy can be transformed from one form to another but cannot be created or destroyed. This law is usually formulated as follows: The rate of change in body E_S[10] is equal to the difference between the rates of E_I and E_O. All of these terms are expressed as energy per unit of time.

E_I primarily consists of the chemical energy from the food and fluids we consume. E_O includes the radiant, conductive, and convective heat lost; any work performed; and the latent heat of evaporation. E_S is the rate of change in the body's macronutrient stores. The energy balance equation ($E_S = E_I - E_O$) is a statement of the principle of energy conservation.

Components of Intake

Energy intake includes 3 major macronutrient groups—carbohydrate, protein, and fat—and a smaller component from alcohol. Once ingested, the net absorption of the major macronutrient groups is variable and incomplete, with fecal losses accounting for ~ 2–10% of gross E_I. The net absorption of dietary energy components varies among individuals and is dependent on the specific foods eaten, how they are prepared, and intestinal factors.

The metabolizable energy (hereafter referred to as E_I) of a diet represents the difference between the absolute energy of ingested substrates and the energy losses found in feces and urine. Commonly used energy densities for carbohydrate (4 kcal/g, 17 kJ/g), protein (4 kcal/g, 17 kJ/g), and fat (9 kcal/g, 38 kJ/g) represent population averages for metabolizable energy, which is the amount of fuel actually available to cells for conducting biological processes.

Digestibility depends on the composition of the food item and on its content of fiber and other indigestible components. Such components can mechanically limit the access of digestive enzymes to food that would potentially be digestible. For example, nuts and other plant materials have cell walls that cannot be digested by gut enzymes, and they thereby protect the cell contents from digestion if not masticated sufficiently to disrupt the cell structure. These effects can have a large impact on the absorption of ingested macronutrients. The variability in absorptive efficiency depends on many additional factors (eg, gut flora, food preparation, diet composition), which may explain the individual differences in metabolizable E_I.

Components of Expenditure (EO)

Absorbed carbohydrates, proteins, and fats are transformed in vivo to substrates that can ultimately either be oxidized to produce metabolically useful energy that drives biological processes or they may be stored. The rate of whole-body energy expenditure, or E_O, varies within a 24-h period and across the life span. Expended energy reflects fuels metabolized for growth, body maintenance needs, physical activity, pregnancy and lactation, and many other processes.

The main energy expenditure terms are REE, TEF, and AEE. REE is the rate of energy expenditure at rest and comprises approximately two-thirds of E_O. REE varies between and within individuals depending on body size, body composition, and recent energy imbalance. Greater total tissue mass increases REE, and the contribution of lean tissue is greater than fat tissue. Moreover, within lean tissue, high metabolic organs such as the brain, heart, kidney, and liver contribute disproportionately to REE. There is also a large variability in REE (~ 250 kcal/d, ~ 1000 kJ/d) that is not explained by differences in body composition.

The TEF is the obligatory energy expenditure that is associated with digestion and processing of ingested foods. Diet composition has a strong effect on TEF. There is a hierarchy of macronutrient effects on the magnitude of TEF, with isocaloric amounts of protein > carbohydrate > fat. Normally, TEF is assumed to be a fixed percentage of E_I, but variation between and within individuals occurs. AEE is the energy expenditure rate during activity and can be further partitioned into exercise energy expenditure and nonexercise activity thermogenesis.

Components of Storage

Triglycerides, which are present within adipose tissue, are the body's major fuel reserve. A lean adult has ~ 35 billion adipocytes, each containing ~ 0.4–0.6 μ g triglyceride and totaling 130,000 kcal stored energy. An extremely obese adult can have 4 times as many adipocytes (140 billion), each containing twice as much lipid (0.8–1.2 μ g triglyceride) and totaling ~ 1 million kcal stored energy.

E_S reflects net changes in the body mass of carbohydrate, protein, and fat. Carbohydrate is stored mainly in the form of intracellular glycogen in skeletal muscle and liver. The total mass of glycogen is relatively small, several hundred grams, and turnover is rapid; maximal amounts are observed in the postmeal state. Water is weakly bonded to glycogen so that glycogen's synthesis and catabolism also involve alterations in fluid balance. Body protein takes many specific forms and, as with glycogen, is associated with water but at a lower value per gram. Lipid in the form of triglyceride is the largest source of stored energy in most adults and has no water associated with it.

Any imbalance between the intake and utilization of these macronutrients will lead to an alteration in body composition. The energy stored per unit body weight of carbohydrate, fat, and protein varies considerably, especially when accounting for the associated intracellular water. Furthermore, dietary carbohydrate intake has an impact on renal sodium excretion, which results in changes in extracellular fluid. Therefore, changes in body weight are expected when the macronutrient composition of the diet is altered, even when the energy content of the diet is held constant.

The long-term stability of body weight is often considered a marker of zero E_S, and thus energy balance. However, changes in body weight also include changes in body water, which may be variable, and therefore weight change may not directly represent energy imbalances, particularly over the short term.

Energy Expenditure Measurement

Measurement of energy expenditure in humans is required to assess metabolic needs, fuel utilisation, and the relative thermic effect of different food, drink, drug and emotional components. Indirect and direct calorimetric and non-calorimetric methods for measuring energy expenditure are reviewed, and their relative value for measurement in the laboratory and field settings is assessed. Where high accuracy is required and sufficient resources are available, an open-circuit indirect calorimeter can be used. Open-circuit indirect calorimeters can employ a mask, hood, canopy or room/chamber for collection of expired air. For short-term measurements, mask, hood or canopy systems suffice. Chamber-based systems are more accurate for the long-term measurement of specified activity patterns but behaviour constraints mean they do not reflect real life. Where resources are limited and optimum precision can be sacrificed, flexible total collection systems and non-calorimetric methods are potentially useful if the limitations of these methods are appreciated. The use of the stable isotope technique, doubly labelled water, enables total daily energy expenditure to be measured accurately in free-living subjects. The factorial method for combining activity logs and data on the energy costs of activities can also provide detailed information on free-living subjects.

There are three components to total energy expenditure (TEE) in humans: basal metabolic rate (BMR), thermic effect of food and the energy expenditure of activity (activity thermogenesis). BMR is the energy expended when an individual is lying at complete rest, in the morning after sleep in the post-absorptive state. In individuals with sedentary occupations basal metabolic rate accounts for approximately 60% of the total daily energy expenditure and is highly predicted by lean body mass within and across species. Resting energy expenditure, in general, is within 10% of the BMR and is measured in subjects at complete rest in the post- absorptive state. Thermic effect of food is the increase in energy expenditure associated with digestion, absorption and storage of food, and accounts for approximately 10% of the total daily energy expenditure; many believe there exist facultative as well as fixed components. Activity thermogenesis is the thermogenesis that accompanies physical activities and, therefore, can be divided into exercise and non-exercise activity thermogenesis (NEAT). Most individuals do not partake in purposeful sporting exercise and so their exercise-related activity thermogenesis is zero; for those who do exercise regularly, exercise- related energy expenditure is generally ,10% of the total daily energy expenditure. NEAT or the 'energy expenditure of spontaneous physical activity' encompasses the combined energy costs of the physical activities of daily living, fidgeting, spontaneous muscle contraction and maintaining posture when not recumbent, and accounts for the remainder of the total daily energy expenditure for most individuals. Other thermogenic variables may also need to be considered, such as the energetic costs of altered temperature, medications and emotion.

Each of these components of energy expenditure is highly variable and the total effect of these variances determines the variability in daily energy expenditure between individuals. Also, measurements of energy expenditure can be used to assess the relative thermic effects of different foods, nutrient compositions, beve- rages, medications and psychological components.

Description of Methods

Energy expenditure can be measured using one of the three approaches:

- In *indirect calorimetry*, oxygen consumption and carbon dioxide production is measured and converted to energy expenditure using formulae.
- In *direct calorimetry,* the rate of heat loss from the subject to the calorimeter is measured.
- A number of *non-calorimetric* techniques have been used to predict the energy expenditure by extrapolation from physiological measurements and observations.

The accuracy, reproducibility and reliability of the measurements obtained using these various techniques vary enormously as the complexity and cost of the techniques themselves. The techniques are summarised in table.

Indirect Calorimetry

There are five principal approaches to the measurement of energy expenditure using indirect calorimetry.

Total Collection Systems

Here, expired air is collected in either an airtight rigid structure or a portable flexible bag.

Rigid Total Collection System

The Tissot Gasometer is an example of a rigid total collection system. It comprises a 100 – 1000 litre capacity inverted glass bell fitted with an internal circulation fan suspended over water. The bell is emptied of air. The subject then expires through a mouthpiece and a non- return valve into the bell, which gradually fills with expired air and progressively rises above the water seal. The height reached by the bell is recorded every minute for up to 2 hours and the composition of expired air is periodically measured from the bell to determine oxygen consumption and carbon dioxide production.

Flexible Total Collection System

The Douglas bag is an example of a flexible total collection system. It comprises a polyvinyl chloride (or other leak-proof material) bag of typically 100 – 150 litre capacity. The top of the bag is connected by tubing to a three-way valve which may be rotated to either seal the bag, admit atmospheric air or admit expired air via tubing attached to a respiratory valve. To use this approach, the three-way valve is first rotated to open the circuit to atmospheric air, the bag is rolled up to expel its contents and the three-way valve then rotated to seal the bag. The subject breathes through the mouthpiece and the three-way valve is rotated to allow the expired air for 10 – 20 minutes. After the timed collection period, the three-way valve is turned to seal the bag. An alternative valve system employs two valves, one at the mouthpiece and the other proximal to the bag. Several bags can be used to prolong the total measurement period. After collection of the expired air, the volume of the expired air in the bag is measured (for example using a mass flow meter) and a sample is analysed to determine oxygen and carbon dioxide concentrations. Under optimal conditions the error of energy expenditure measurements undertaken with Douglas bags may be very small (,3%) but can increase substantially if the equipment is poorly maintained, the volume, oxygen and carbon dioxide measurements inaccurate and the operator untrained or unskilled.

Open-circuit Indirect Calorimeter Systems

Open-circuit systems can be used to record energy expenditure over several hours or days depending upon the configuration selected and the experimental requirements. In an open-circuit system, the subject inspires air and the expired gases are then analysed. There are two types of open-circuit systems: Ventilated open-circuit systems where a subject breathes into a container through which air is drawn, and expiratory collection systems where a subject inspires from the atmosphere and expires via a non-return valve into a measurement unit.

Ventilated Open-circuit Systems

In general, ventilated open-circuit systems comprise components to collect and mix expired air, measure flow rate, analyse gas concentrations and pump air through the system.

The method of collecting expired air varies considerably. The least complex approach is for expired air to be collected using a mouthpiece, mask, transparent hood or canopy. Measurements can be performed for up to several hours. The most more complex approach is for the subject to be placed inside a room/chamber of known volume in which there are often sophisticated sensing devices to quantify physical activity. Using a room or chamber, measurements can be performed for up to several days.

Regardless of how the expired air is collected, the basic components of ventilated open-circuit indirect calorimeters are similar. Expired air is drawn out of the collection device using a pump; it is critical to measure this flow rate accurately. The expired air is then mixed using a fan and mixing chamber, and a sample of the expired air is dried and analysed for oxygen and carbon dioxide concentrations. Oxygen is generally analysed by using paramagnetic analysers and carbon dioxide by using infrared analysers; alternatively, a mass spectrometer can be used to measure the gas concentrations. Burning known masses of chemical standards, such as butane or ethanol, within the system and ascertaining what proportion of the burned mass is detected by the calorimeter verifies the precision of these calorimeters. Ventilated open-circuit indirect calorimeters have precision to within 0.5 – 2% of actual.

Table: Summary of techniques used to measure energy expenditure in humans.

Approach	Type of calorimeter	Basal metabolic rate	Resting energy expenditure	Thermic effect of food	Energy expenditure of specific activities	Total daily energy expenditure
Indirect calorimete	Room open-circuit	Yes	Yes	Yes	Yes	Yes (confined subject)
	Hood/canopy open-circuit	Yes	Yes	Yes	Yes	No
	Open-circuit expiratory collection	Yes*	Yes*	Yes*	Yes	Yes*
	Doubly labelled water	No	No	No	No	yes
	Total collection Douglas bag	Yes	Yes	Yes*	Yes	No
Direct calorimeter		Yes	Yes	Yes	Yes	Yes
Non-calorimetric methods		No	No	No	No	Estimated

Depending on the software, air mixing and room volume, response time for a room or chamber system can vary from ~5 to 30 minutes; for a ventilated hood or canopy,~2 minutes and for a mask or mouthpiece <30 seconds. Hood/canopy/mask-based systems are often configured as a 'metabolic cart' whereby the equipment could be readily moved on a wheeled cart. Finally, it is important that inspired carbon dioxide should not exceed 1% as concentrations in excess of this may increase respiratory effort.

Expiratory Collection Open-circuit Systems

There are several expiratory collection open-circuit systems. The advantage of this approach is that the calorimeter can be designed as a portable device so that energy expenditure can be measured in free-living individuals. In general, these devices comprise a mouth- piece or a mask connected to a one-way valve whereby expired air enters the instrument. The flow rate of expired air through the valve is measured and a small proportion of the expired air is diverted to a gas storage reservoir that is analysed at the end of each measurement period. Measurements can be carried out using such instruments intermittently for up to 2 days. Various modifications have been applied to this principle; for example, by having air drawn through the system at a fixed rate. Technological advance has resulted in the design of more precise, robust and dependable portable calorimeters that are likely to provide useful field data in the future.

Confinement System (Respiratory Chambers)

The subject is placed inside a gas-tight sealed container of known volume (e.g. 16 m^3) and oxygen consumption and carbon dioxide production are estimated from changes in the concentrations of these gases in chamber air over time. The period of observation may be prolonged by periodically flushing the chamber with fresh air. A number of confinement systems have been constructed with errors of ~2% and response times of ~50 minutes. Currently, confinement systems are rarely used.

Closed-circuit Systems

Closed-circuit systems consist of a sealed respiratory gas circuit in which gaseous concentrations are measured over time. In one conformation, expired air was drawn from a sealed 5 m^3 chamber. Carbon dioxide and water vapour were absorbed and then oxygen was reintroduced into the air stream, which re-entered the chamber. Energy expenditure was calculated from the quantities of carbon dioxide absorbed and oxygen re-introduced. A small-scale application of this approach was to use a spirometer. A spirometer consists of an oxygen-containing bell from which the subject inspires; expired carbon dioxide and water vapour are absorbed before the expired air is reintroduced to the bell. The bell is suspended over water so that its height descends at a rate proportional to oxygen consumption. Closed-circuit systems are rarely used at present.

Body Composition in an Athlete

Body composition is a method of describing what the body is made of. It includes fat, protein, minerals and body water. It also describes weight more accurately than BMI. Body composition analysis can accurately show changes in fat mass, muscle mass, and body fat percentage. This can help validate services like personal training, patient care, and corporate wellness. The assessment of an athlete's physiology is a key skill for the applied exercise physiologist as it allows for the planning of training and competition strategy. One key aspect of this assessment is the analysis of his/her body composition.

Body composition analysis involves division of the total body mass into its constituent parts, or compartments. This allows an athlete, coach or team to monitor the physiological make-up of the athlete, to determine, for instance, whether training or rehabilitation following injury is proving effective. Wang and colleagues described the human body as comprising five levels of organisation moving from micro (Level 1) to macro. Models of body composition are broadly based on the number of compartments between which they differentiate with the two-compartment model the most simple of these (fat and fat-free mass) and the multi-compartment model (mass and atomic/molecular composition) the most complicated. The full range of models of body composition including the methods of assessing them are presented in table.

There are numerous methods of measuring body composition, characterised as direct, indirect or doubly indirect, each presenting its own advantages and limitations. Direct methods involve dissecting a cadaver and then chemically deriving the amount of each individual tissue that is present, whereas indirect methods use imaging to quantify the amounts of each tissue present. Finally, doubly indirect methods use measurements taken on the body, in conjunction with data obtained from previous studies using direct methods to estimate the amount of each tissue present based on a variety of different equations. These are discussed in greater detail later on. Direct methods, whilst being the most accurate, are never used in an applied setting as they involve dissection and chemical analysis meaning they are therefore not practical for use with athletes. As a result indirect methods are much more commonly used. Some indirect methods, such as Magnetic Resonance Imaging (MRI) and Computed Topography (CT) are in contrast not readily available, and therefore not often used in an applied setting as they are costly and involve specialist equipment or personnel. An indirect method that is used in an applied setting is dual-energy x-ray absorptiometry, and this is discussed in greater depth below. A major limitation of indirect methods is that their underpinning assumptions are based on a number of early studies involving direct methods, These assumptions include that fat storage is the same in all individuals, whereas it is very different between males and females as well as between different ethnic groups, regardless of individual variations in storage sites. Another major limitation is that these methods assume that fat is of homogenous density.

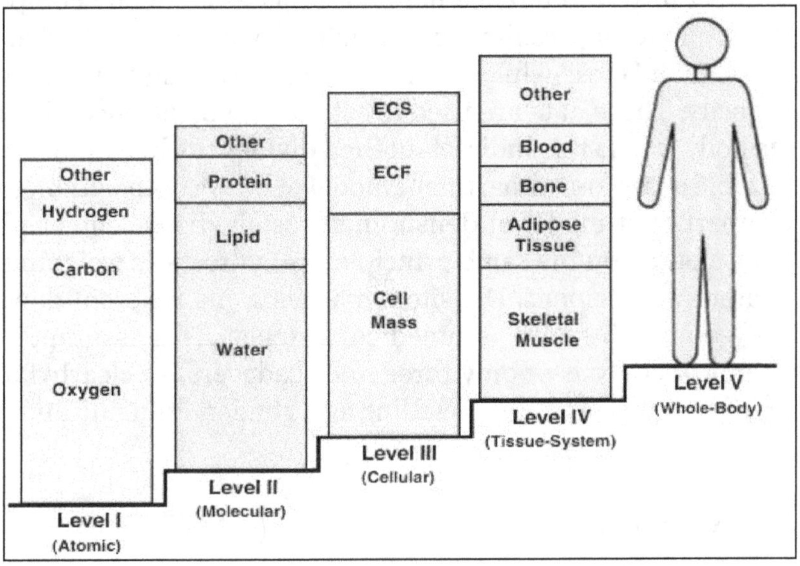

The five levels of human body composition.

Table: Models of body composition analysis and examples of compartmental break-down and analysis techniques.

Number of Compartments	Example of compartmental breakdown	Example of analysis technique(s)
Two	Fat & fat-free mass	Hydrodensitometry (ID), skinfold formulae (DID)
Three	Bone mineral, fat & mineral free, fat-free mass	DXA (ID)
Four	Bone mineral, fat, protein & water	DXA (ID), hydrodensitometry (ID) & a measure of total body water (DID)
Five	Bone mineral, fat, protein, ICW & ECW	DXA (ID) & whole-body counting or isotope dilution (ID)
Multi	Mass and atomic/molecular composition of individual tissues or organs	CT, MRI (ID)

These limitations are evident in all indirect and doubly indirect methods as they are not measuring the actual amount of each different tissue; instead they rely on making educated estimations based on normative data from cadaver studies by. Finally, doubly indirect methods, such as anthropometry and bioelectrical impedance, whilst cost effective and widely used in the public health and fitness industries, should be used with caution in athletic populations as they demonstrate poor accuracy and replicability.

A number of indirect methods are used in an applied setting and these are outlined below before focusing on dual-energy x-ray absorptiometry.

Densitometry

A traditional indirect in vivo reference method for assessing body composition is hydrostatic weighing. Based on Archimedes' principle, body volume is calculated taking into account mass in air, mass while submerged and exhaling maximally underwater and the water density. These data are used to estimate body density which in turn predicts percentage body fat. As this indirect method divides the body into fat and fat- free mass it is an example of a two-compartment model of body composition. Another widely used two- compartment model of densitometry is air-displacement plethysmogrophy. This method is based on the same principles as hydrostatic weighing but employs air instead of water displacement. Densitometry has some inherent flaws, principally that fat and fat-free mass have an assumed consistency. This assumption however is based on the chemical analysis of only three male cadavers, so clearly fails to account for a number of influencing variables including age, gender, ethnicity and disease states at death.

Bioelectrical Impedance

Perhaps the most common method of body composition, bioelectrical impedance is widely used at most leisure centres and gyms. Another two-compartment model, bioelectrical impedance makes use of the different electrical conductivity of fat and fat-free mass. Due to its high water content, fat-free mass conducts a small electrical current, whereas anhydrous fat mass provides resistance and therefore does not act as a conductor. An impedance value is established, and taking into account mass, stature and water content fat mass is predicted. As a doubly indirect method, bioelectrical impedance is however, quite unreliable as it is based on a number of assumptions and is greatly affected by hydration status.

Anthropometry

Anthropometry is the measurement of lengths, circumferences and skinfold thicknesses of the body. Using equations developed by and estimated body density can be converted into body fat percentage. Skinfolds are a useful measure for coaches to employ as they are quick to measure and make use of inexpensive equipment. However obtaining accurate measures requires a degree of skill from the operator that is not often demonstrated, and as are other indirect methods, are based on a series of assumptions that do not universally apply across populations.

References

- Current-knowledge-and-new-challenges-in-exercise-immunology: he.kendallhunt.com, Retrieved 19 April, 2019
- About-kinesiology: aka.asn.au, Retrieved 23 June, 2019
- Neuroplasticity: scienceforsport.com, Retrieved 18 July, 2019
- 3-key-principles-of-kinesiology: medium.com, Retrieved 15 March, 2019
- Energy-balance, sports-and-everyday-life-food-and-drink-food-and-cooking: encyclopedia.com, Retrieved 16 April, 2019
- The-Measurement-of-Body-Composition-in-an-Athletic-Population-The-Importance-of-DXA-275512032: researchgate.net, Retrieved 14 June, 2019

3

The Physics of Sports

Use of physics in sports is termed as physics of sports. It is a vast subject that branches out into sports biomechanics, kinematics of human motion, linear kinetics in sports, angular kinematics, fluid mechanics, sport aerodynamics, impulse and momentum, etc., which have been thoroughly discussed in this chapter.

Sports Biomechanics

All life forms on earth are subjected to gravity. How the form, function and motion of these biological systems are affected directly or indirectly by gravity has been a subject of scientific study over centuries. It started with the development of mechanics that were concerned with the behavior of physical bodies when subjected to forces or displacements, and the subsequent effect of the bodies on their environment. More than 3000 years ago Babylonian astronomers studied the problem of planetary positions. The Renaissance astronomer Nicolaus Copernicus published his heliocentric theory in 1543, which was in contrast to the widely accepted geocentric system model popular during the 13th–17th centuries that had been proposed by Aristotle and Claudius Ptolemy. During the early modern period, renowned scientists, including Galileo, Kepler and Newton, laid the foundation of classical mechanics. worked theoretically and experimentally on the motions of bodies, particularly of falling bodies. empirically discovered his laws of planetary motion which gave an approximate description of the motion of planets around the sun and provided one of the foundations for Isaac Newton's theory of universal gravitation. In 1687 Isaac Newton used the newly developed mathematics of calculus to give a detailed mathematical explanation of mechanics and published his classic Philosophiae Naturalis Principia Mathematica. In this three-volume publication he formulated the law of universal gravitation and the three laws of motion which can be applied to the motion of planets in the heavens and all forms of movements on earth. Since all life forms on earth are under the influence of universal gravitation, there is no doubt that mechanics not only governs the motions of lifeless objects, but also affects the form, motion and function of the biological systems on earth. The mechanical interactions within the biological systems and with the environment received attention from early scholars as well as from scientists of the present day. Their efforts on the discovery of these mechanical interactions have come to form a discipline of research called biomechanics.

Biomechanics is the study of continuum mechanics (that is, the study of loads, motion, stress, and strain of solids and fluids) of biological systems and the mechanical effects on the body's movement, size, shape and structure. Mechanical influence on biological systems can be found at multiple levels, from molecular and cellular, all the way up to the tissue, organ and system level. Therefore, the study of biomechanics of humans ranges from the inner workings of a cell, the mechanical properties of soft and hard tissues, to the development and movement of the neuromusculoskeletal system of the body. Molecular biomechanics refers to the study of how mechanical forces and deformation affect the conformation, binding/reaction, function and transport of biomolecules, such as DNA, RNA and proteins, and how mechanobiochemistry couples in biomolecular motors and ion channel flows, etc. Cellular biomechanics is concerned with the study of how cells sense mechanical forces or deformations, and transduce them into biological responses, especially for the study of how mechanical forces alter cell growth, differentiation, movement, signal transduction, protein secretion and transport, gene expression and regulation. The properties of living tissues are affected by applied loads and deformations, and tissue biomechanics is mainly concerned with the growth and remodeling of tissues as a response to applied mechanical stimuli. For example, the effects of elevated blood pressure on the mechanics of the arterial wall, and the behavior of cardiomyocytes within a heart with a cardiac infarct, have been widely regarded as instances in which living tissue is remodeled as a direct consequence of applied loads. Another example is Wolff's law of bone remodeling, developed by Julius Wolff (1836–1902) in the 19th century. Wolff's laws states that the internal architecture of the trabecular bone and the external cortical bone in a healthy person or animal will adapt to the loads placed on the bone and it will remodel itself over time to become stronger to resist that type of loading. The converse is also true. If the loading on a bone decreases, the bone will become weaker owing to turnover and a lack of stimulus for continued remodeling that is required to maintain bone mass.

At the system level, mechanical factors also affect the form, performance and function of the musculoskeletal system. Human movement is achieved by a complex and highly coordinated mechanical interaction between bones, muscles, ligaments and joints within the musculoskeletal system under the control of the nervous system. Muscles generate tensile forces and apply moments at joints with short lever arms in order to provide static and dynamic stability of the body under gravitational and other loads while regularly performing precise limb control. Any injury or lesion of any of the individual elements of the musculoskeletal system will change the mechanical interaction and cause degradation, instability or disability of movement. On the other hand, proper modification, manipulation and control of the mechanical environment can help prevent injury, correct abnormality, and speed healing and rehabilitation. Therefore, understanding the biomechanics and loading of each element is helpful for studying disease etiology, making treatment decisions and evaluating the effects of treatment. However, because of ethical considerations and technological limitations, direct measurement of the forces transmitted in the human body is possible only in exceptional circumstances, such as through instrumented implants. A further challenge is the redundant nature of the musculoskeletal system. In the human body there are more joints and muscles than are necessary for performing our daily motor tasks. Therefore, a certain task can be achieved by more than one musculoskeletal strategy. However, this compensatory mechanism is essential for coping with the consequences of injuries or diseases to the musculoskeletal system, but it makes it difficult to determine the internal forces noninvasively.

Currently, combining noninvasive measurements of the movement, such as the position of segments and the strain on force-measuring instruments, with computer graphics-based anatomical modeling is a useful approach to estimating these loadings. In this approach it is essential to integrate the techniques of motion analysis and medical imaging. They include measuring human motion and external loads, developing three-dimensional (3D) computer graphics-based biomechanical models based on medical imaging, calculating internal forces and validating the results. A validated 3D computer biomechanical model can then be applied to the simulation of various movements and surgical procedures. A recording of an electromyogram (EMG) of the active muscles can further be used to understand the muscle activity during human movement. However, developing a precise and noninvasive method for measuring the internal force within the human body for clinical and other purposes still remains a great challenge in the field of human biomechanics and motion analysis.

Kinematics of Human Motion

Many of us have been enthralled while watching world-class gymnasts perform seemingly impossible maneuvers on television, or been thrilled at a stellar dance performance. These events involve varying degrees of human motion to execute them.

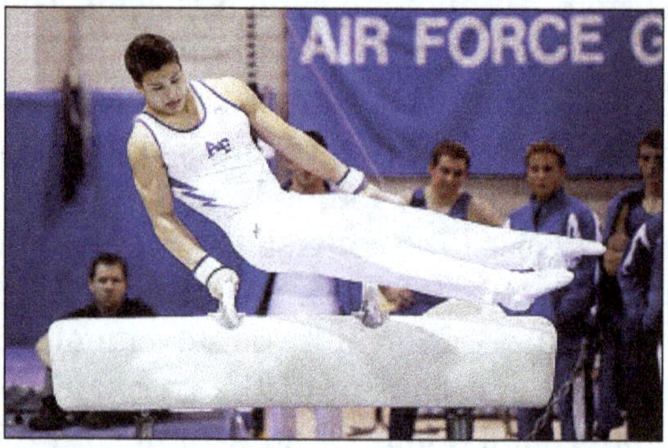

Gymnast in motion on the pommel horse.

Newton's first law states that, in general, an object at rest stays in rest, while an object in motion stays in motion. This is also known as inertia and definitely applies to the human body and human motion.

The study of human motion is a branch of biomechanics known as kinematics. Kinematics specifically studies just pure motion and not the actual forces which cause the motion. There are several types of motions exhibited by the human body.

Translatory and Rotational Motion

Most human motion involves a combination of two types of motion, translatory motion, also known as linear motion, and rotational motion, also known as angular motion. Think of a long jumper sprinting toward the sandy pit. He is exhibiting translatory motion as he runs in a straight line. Then he takes off and swings his arms to try and stay airborne, which is a form of rotational motion. Together, the combined movements are general motion.

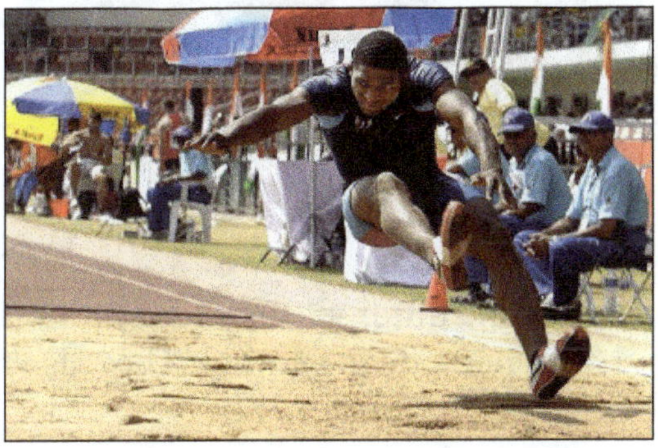

A long jumper exhibits general motion.

Three Planes of Motion

The human body is three-dimensional (it has height, width, and depth), although it often just moves in two dimensions in what is known as planar motion. While space is three-dimensional, a plane is simply a surface of two-dimensions that extends to infinity (forever.) Therefore, planar motion is motion that involves only two of the three dimensions. The human body moves through three distinct planes:

- Frontal Plane - Did you ever have to do jumping jacks in gym class? Those were an example of movement in the frontal plane. With jumping jacks, there is both side-to-side movement of the arms and legs and also an up-and-down movement; however, there is no third movement of forward-and-backward.
- Sagittal Plane - Movement in the sagittal plane involves bending forward and backward along with up and down; however, there is very little side-to side motion. These movements tend to be the most common used when exercising. Lunges and curls are two notable examples.
- Transverse Plane - Movement in the transverse plane tends to be a little more complex because it often involves rotational movements. A common example would be to do lunges while holding a medicine ball, but this time step diagonally

instead of forward. First step diagonally to the left. Then, return the feet to the original position. Then, step diagonally to the right. Do you see how this would involve a twisting, or rotational, motion of the body? Within this plane, the body moves up/down, forward/backward, and side to side.

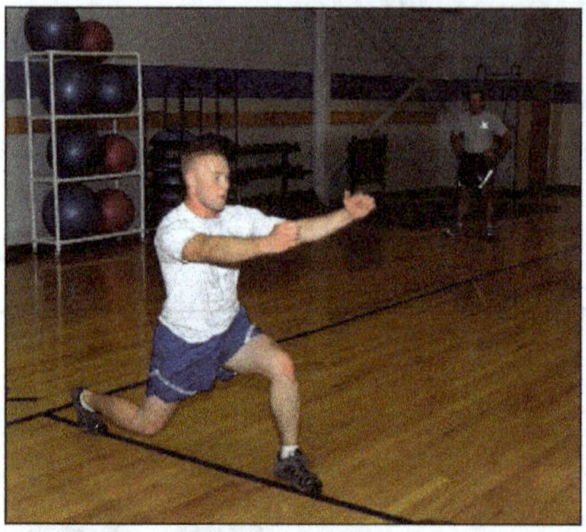

A lunge in the sagittal plane.

Anatomical Terms for Motion

Now let us expound on some of the different terms for motion. These movements can be at angles, in circles, and from one side to another. They also range from the head and neck to the torso and the limbs.

Flexion vs. Extension

Flexion is simply a decreasing of the angle between two given body parts. Extension is the opposite, and thus is the increasing of the angle. During a bicep curl, you would bring your palm and the dumbbell toward your shoulder, which would decrease the angle between your upper arm and your forearm. This is an example of flexion, or more familiarly stated, you are flexing your muscle. When you lower the dumbbell back down, you increase the angle between your upper arm and your lower arm. This would be an example of extension.

Linear Kinetics in Sports

Newton's Laws of Motion

Newton's Three Laws of Motion explain how forces create motion in sport. These laws are usually referred to as the Laws of Inertia, Acceleration, and Reaction.

- Law of Inertia - Newton's First Law of inertia states that objects tend to resist changes in their state of motion. An object in motion will tend to stay in motion and an object at rest will tend to stay at rest unless acted upon by a force. Example - The body of a player quickly sprinting down the field will tend to want to retain that motion unless muscular forces can overcome this inertia or a skater gliding on ice will continue gliding with the same speed and in the same direction, barring the action of an external force.

- Law of Acceleration - Newton's Second Law precisely explains how much motion a force creates. The acceleration (tendency of an object to change speed or direction) an object experiences is proportional to the size of the force and inversely proportional to the object's mass (F = ma). Example - When a ball is thrown, kicked, or struck with an implement, it tends to travel in the direction of the line of action of the applied force. Similarly, the greater the amount of force applied, the greater the speed the ball has. If a player improves leg strength through training while maintaining the same body mass, they will have an increased ability to accelerate the body using the legs, resulting in better agility and speed.
- Law of Reaction - The Third Law states that for every action (force) there is an equal and opposite reaction force. This means that forces do not act alone, but occur in equal and opposite pairs between interacting bodies. Example - The force created by the legs "pushing" against the ground results in ground reaction forces in which the ground "pushes back" and allows the player to move across the court (As the Earth is much more massive than the player, the player accelerates and moves rapidly, while the Earth does not really accelerate or move at all). This action-reaction also occurs at impact with the ball as the force applied to the ball is matched with an equal and opposite force applied to the racket/body.

Gravitational Force

Newton's Law of Universal Gravitation is used to explain gravitational force. This law states that every massive particle in the universe attracts every other massive particle with a force which is directly proportional to the product of their masses and inversely proportional to the square of the distance between them. This general, physical law was derived from observations made by induction. Another way, more modern, way to state the law is: 'every point mass attracts every single other point mass by a force pointing along the line intersecting both points. The force is proportional to the product of the two masses and inversely proportional to the square of the distance between the point masses'.

Gravitational force surrounds us. It is what decides how much we weigh and how far a basketball will travel when thrown before it returns to the surface. The gravitational force on Earth is equal to the force the Earth exerts on you. At rest, on or near the surface of the Earth, the gravitational force equals your weight. On a different astronomical body like Venus or the Moon, the acceleration of gravity is different than on Earth, so if you were to stand on a scale, it would show you that you weigh a different amount than on Earth.

When two objects are gravitational locked, their gravitational force is centered in an area that is not at the center of either object, but at the barycenter of the system. The principle is similar to that of a see-saw. If two people of very different weights sit on opposite sides of the balance point, the heavier one must sit closer to the balance point so that they can equalize each others mass. For instance, if the heavier person weighs twice as much as the lighter one, they must sit at only half the distance from the fulcrum. The balance point is the center of mass of the see-saw, just as the barycenter is the balance point of the Earth-Moon system. This point that actually moves around the Sun in the orbit of the Earth, while the Earth and Moon each move around the barycenter, in their orbits.

Since gravity is a universal force that is always upon us it must be considered in regard to how it affects human movement.

How gravity affects human movement in general: Gravity actually causes the body to move by its constant pull on the body's Center of Mass (also referred to as the Center of Gravity). The Earth's gravitational force always pulls at a body's Center Of Mass (COM), whether it is the human body, a bowling ball, a car, etc. The human body moves when the COM shifts away from the intersection point of three cardinal planes (Frontal, Sagittal, Transverse) of the body. This shift causes torque to be produced about the joints thus causing the body to move (locomotion).

When we are considering dynamic movement such as sprinting we can either use gravity to our advantage or fight against it. This becomes extremely important when we need to accelerate and decelerate. For maximum acceleration we need to shift the upper-body forward with as significant of a lean as possible. This will cause the COM to shift forward and away from the body. Since gravity always pulls at an object's COM when body mass is manipulated in this manner gravity will pull the body forward and assist us. A great example of this is when sprinters come out of the blocks and are in a "drive phase" posture.

A sprinter will not remain in this posture over the course of the sprint because once inertia is overcome this is not a mechanically efficient position to be in. If the same sprinter is in an upright body position and the body's COM is close to the body then gravity is pulling the body straight down and working against the sprinter. This is a very common mistake that junior athletes make when trying to get a good jump and produce maximum speed as quickly as possible.

How pronounced should the forward upper-body lean be? As pronounced as possible without losing balance. As with all sports movement there is a "point of diminishing returns" with regard to moving body segment mass at which body control and balance are adversely affected. When sprinting we want to manipulate body mass and maximize range of motion about the hips and shoulders without adversely affecting performance.

The position of the head plays a significant role in upper-body lean. The head is actually a major balance factor. For maximum upper-body lean the head should be DOWN. Very important to note here that by the head being down we do not want the chin tucked tightly to the chest, but rather the head should be down and FORWARD. For proper down position of the head the athlete should see the ground 3 or 4 yards ahead of him, not directly under him. With the head in the proper position the COM is extended slightly further and this small extension can make a difference.

Centre of Gravity

The centre of gravity is the point at which gravity appears to be acting upon an object, this is for the most part the same as the point around which the mass of an object or person is equally distributed in all directions. For the average human, the centre of gravity is at the centre of the pelvis when they are standing in the anatomical position. The centre of gravity shifts slightly upwards for males due to their larger shoulder mass, but centre of gravity is always athlete specific. This means that an athlete with larger legs will have a lower centre of gravity unless their upper body is also large and balances the mass.

The centre of gravity moves according to the athlete's body position. For example, in the runner in the image above, his centre of gravity is in the lower region of the pelvis and in front of his body, because his upper body is leaning forwards. Having the centre of gravity lower and in front of his lower body is advantageous for acceleration.

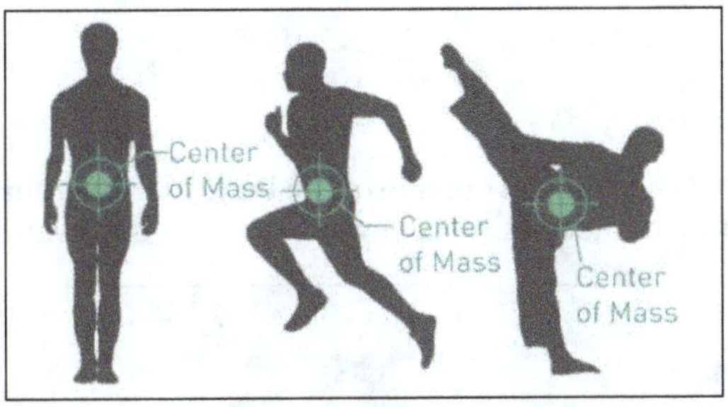

The centre of gravity (COG) in the anatomical position, while running upright, and while completing a kick in martial arts (left to right).

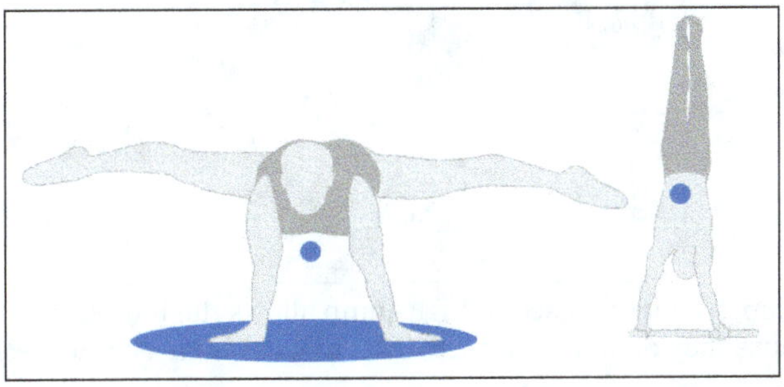

The COG in 2 gymnastics poses. Notice that the one on the left is outside of the body.

Lowering your centre of gravity also helps to increase stability because it needs to be lifted higher before it moves outside of the base of support. This becomes very useful in combat sports such a jujitsu or sumo wrestling. It is also used by blockers in the NFL or to create a more effective rugby league tackle.

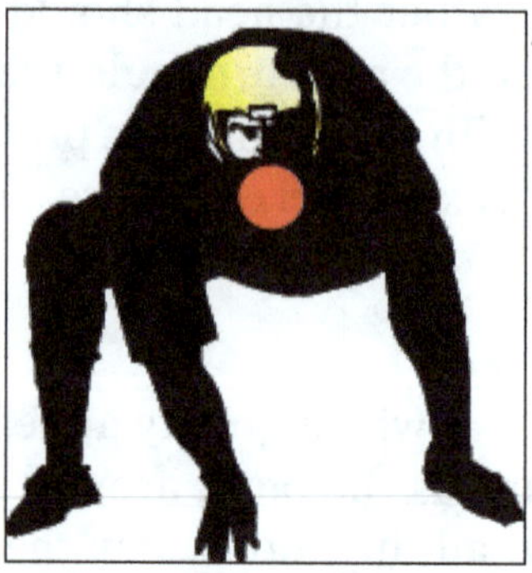

The NFL blocker lowers his COG in order to increase his stability and remain upright while blocking the sacker.

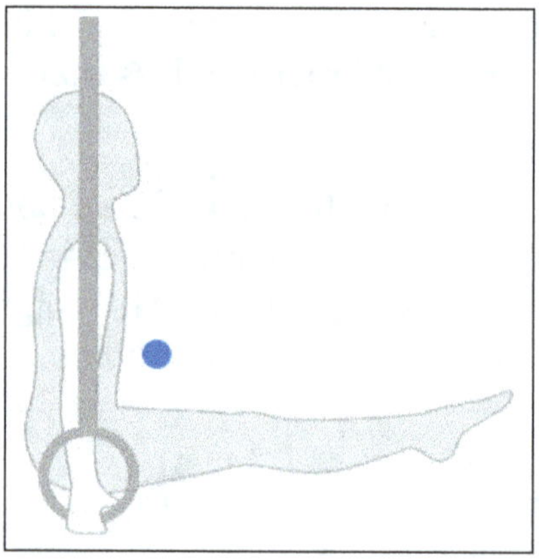

The COG has moved outside of the body in this gymnastics pose because the legs have been pointed forward.

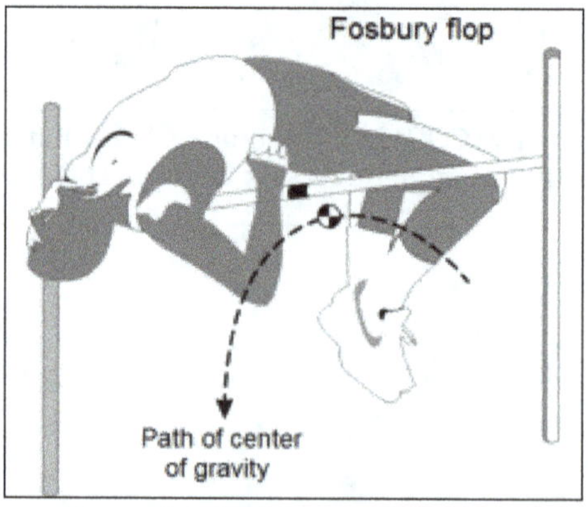

The Fosbury Flop, frequently used in high-jump allows the jumper to go over a higher bar, because they do not need their COG to go as high as other techniques.

Lowering the centre of gravity increases balance and stability in sport. This is why you can change direction faster by bending your legs and getting lower to the ground. It increases your stability, allowing you to adjust to greater force production by the legs.

Principles of Force in Sports

Principles of force offer guidance for teaching sport techniques and leveraging training strategies that require the development of force-pushing or pulling. Force is the product of the mass (weight) and acceleration of an object or person. These principles and examples concern general applications, athlete-produced force and force dissipation.

General Principles of Force

1. Total force (velocity) is the sum of all the forces contributed by each body part. In any explosive skill, each force in sequence should be applied at the peak of the previous force. Examples include throwing a ball and performing a power clean.

2. Force is used more economically when it is applied constantly and evenly. For example, a swimmer moves more efficiently when moving at constant speed and with smooth application of force.

3. All forces should be applied in the intended direction. Deviations from the required line of force waste energy. For example, a runner who points his toes outward or bounces excessively exerts wasted force and energy.

4. Greater velocity is generated if force is applied over a longer distance. For example, an outfielder can generate greater force for throwing to home plate by using a long winding up, rotating the trunk, shifting body weight from the back leg to the front, and following through.

Principles Concerning Athlete-produced Force

1. To achieve maximum force, use larger muscles in the lower body before actions of the trunk and upper body. For example, the force of a punch in boxing or throwing is greater when initiated from the lower body and hips, rather than from the shoulders.

2. Maintain a firm base of support to develop maximum force for throwing and striking. For example, a tennis player can generate a more powerful stroke if the feet are firmly set against the surface of the court.

3. Force generated by muscles can be increased by increasing initial tension before a contraction. This increase in force production is called elastic recoil, or the stretch-shortening cycle. For example, drawing the arm back to pitch a ball or throw a javelin places the muscles of the throwing arm on stretch, increasing the force of contraction upon the initiation of the throw.

4. Executing a follow through at the end of a throwing or striking action maximizes force generation and eliminates the tendency to decelerate prematurely. For example,

reversing the feet at the end of the shot put or discus maximizes acceleration while helping prevent fouling.

Principles Concerning Force Absorption

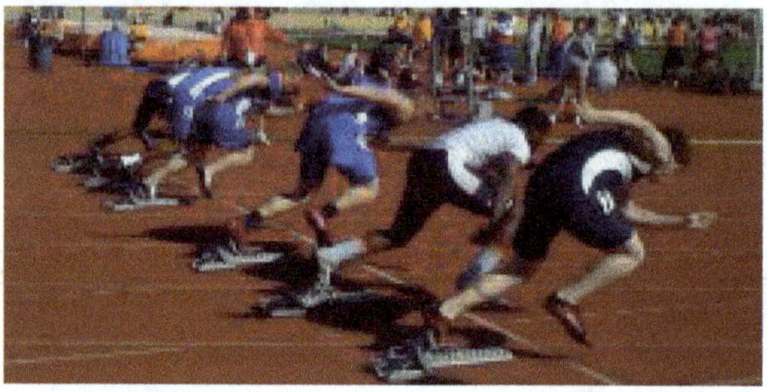

1. The force of a blow can be diminished by distributing the force over a greater time, distance, or area. For example, flexing the joints or rolling on the ground can help an athlete absorb the shock of landing at the end of jump or fall.

2. Transferring momentum from vertical to horizontal can reduce force over a longer time and greater surface area. For example, football players fall and roll to dissipate the force of hitting the ground.

3. Catching objects should be accomplished by extending the arms and fingers, flexing to absorb force and reduce the velocity of the object, and grasping with the fingers to secure the object.

Rate of Force Development (RFD)

The rate of force development (RFD) is a measure of explosive strength, or simply how fast an athlete can develop force – hence the 'rate' of 'force development'. This is defined as the speed at which the contractile elements of the muscle can develop force. Therefore, improving an athlete's RFD may make them more explosive as they can develop larger forces in a shorter period of time. Developing a more explosive athlete may improve their sporting performance. In fact, higher RFDs have been directly linked with better jump, sprint, cycling, weightlifting, and even golf swing performances.

The RFD is commonly believed to be manifested during the stretch-shortening cycle (SSC). Depending upon the duration of the stretch-shortening cycle (SSC), exercises are classified as either slow- (≥250 milliseconds) or fast-SSC (≤250 milliseconds) movements. For example, a countermovement jump (CMJ) is classified as a slow-SSC movement as the duration of the SSC lasts approximately 500 milliseconds. On the other hand, sprinting is classified as a fast-SSC movement as the duration of the SSC lasts between 80-90 milliseconds. Table displays the SSC durations of some common exercises.

Table: SSC durations of common exercises.

Exercise	SSC Duration (Ms)	SSC Classification
Race Walking (14)	270-300	Slow
Sprinting (13)	80-90	Fast
Countermovement Jump (CMJ)(3)	500	Slow
Drop Jump (20cm – 60cm)(15, 16)	130-300	Fast/Slow
Long Jump (17)	140-170	Fast
Multiple Hurdle Jumps (18)	150	Fast

Because the movement is slower, exercises with slow-SSC have a longer timeframe to develop force than those with a fast-SSC, this means slow-SSC exercises can typically create higher peak forces. However, as there is typically less urgency to develop force during the slow-SSC movements, they often do not develop force as quickly as fast-SSC movements. This means that exercises with a slow-SSC produce lower RFDs than fast-SSC movements. Therefore, slow-SSC exercises produce higher peak forces, but lower RFD than fast-SSC movements.

On the other hand, as it takes 140-710 milliseconds to develop peak force during various jump exercises, fast-SSC exercises may struggle to produce peak forces because the SSC simply does not last long enough. Whilst they may not be capable of producing peak forces, they can produce large a RFD due to the speed of the movement.

Table: Differences between force-time characteristics of various exercises.

Exercise	Peak Force (N)	Time to Peak Force (N)	Peak RFD	Time to Peak RFD
Isometric Mid-Thigh pull	3,177	0.25	22,008	0.12
Mid-/Thigh Clean Pull @ 30\\90% of 1RM	2,327	0.25	23,472	0.14
Mid-/Thigh Clean Pull @ 90% of 1RM	1,817	0.15	27,607	0.09
Countermovement Jump (CMJ)	1,449	0.39	12,093	0.26
Squat Jump (SJ)	1,663	0.32	11,529	0.19

Data extracted from experienced male weightlifters Kawamori.

It is suggested that exercises characterised by larger joint displacements (i.e. work through a larger range of movement) are typically categorised as slow-SSC movements. Whereas exercises with smaller joint displacements are commonly referred to as fast-SSC movements. For example, a CMJ (slow-SSC movement) experiences larger joint displacements than sprinting (fast-SSC). This helps to dissociate between what are slow-SSC movements and what are fast-SSC movements when no research has determined what classification they belong too.

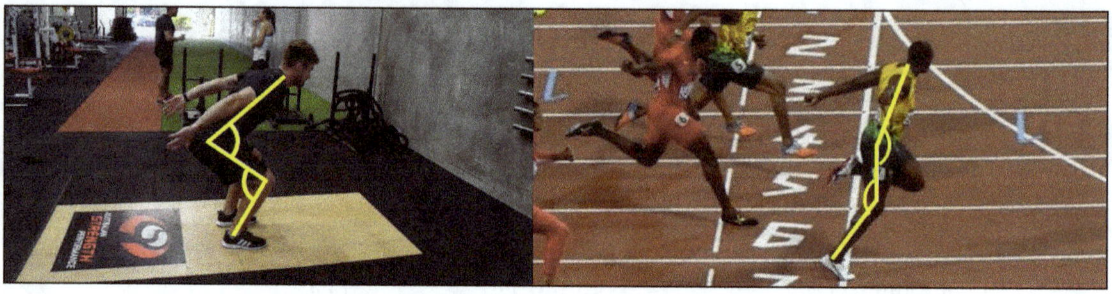

Joint displacement difference between slow-SSC and fast-SSC actions.

What Causes an Increase in Rate of Force Development?

Improvements in RFD are likely to be the result of increases in muscle-tendon stiffness, enhanced muscle force production via changes in muscle fibre type or type area (from type I to type IIA), and increases in neural drive during the early phase of the SSC (<100ms). In contrast, RFD appears to be negatively affected by changes in muscle fibre type (from type IIX to type IIA), and increases in fascicle length (causing reduced muscle stiffness).

Why is the Rate of Force Development Important for Sports?

As power is a key determinant in the performances of many sports, optimising an athlete's explosiveness may be of great importance. Research has identified that the RFD has been directly linked to performances during jumping, weightlifting, cycling, sprinting, and even during the golf swing – suggesting a better RFD can lead to a better athletic performance. Moreover, elite sprinters have been shown to possess greater RFD than well-trained sprinters. Collectively, this information suggests that RFD may be an important contributor to athletic performance.

- RFD linked to better jump, sprint, cycling, weightlifting and golf swing performances.
- Elite-level sprinters have better RFD than well-trained sprinters.
- Power trained athletes have greater RFD than non-power trained athletes.
- Power trained athletes have greater RFD than endurance athletes.

How to Calculate the Rate of Force Development

As RFD is an expression of explosive strength, it is measured in Newtons per second squared ($N \cdot s^{-1}$). The RFD can be calculated for isometric, concentric and eccentric muscle contractions, with the latter two otherwise referred to in the research as the 'positive' and 'negative' acceleration phases of the SSC. In fact, one study suggests that eccentric RFD is a better predictor of jump performance than concentric RFD because it summarises several intrinsic properties of muscle and tendons during a key moment. However, this is yet to be validated by other research.

Multiple measures of RFD have been developed in order to measure various components of performance during both isometric and dynamic movements:

- Average RFD or IES (Index of Explosiveness).
- Time-interval RFD.
- Instantaneous RFD.
- Peak or maximal RFD.
- Time to peak RFD.

Average RFD: This value is identical to the IES discussed by Zatsiorsky, and is calculated by dividing the peak force by the time to achieve peak force. However, this form of measuring average RFD has been shown to have lower levels of reliability in comparison to time-interval RFD and peak RFD. These lower levels of reliability may be associated with each athlete's time to achieve peak force, as not all athletes can achieve peak force in the same time frame. Therefore, measuring RFD using predetermined time-intervals can accommodate for these variances.

How to Calculate Average RFD

Example – Calculating Average RFD:

Average RFD [$N \cdot s^{-1}$] = Peak Force [N]/Time to achieve peak force [s][/toggle]

Time-Interval RFD: Though this measure of RFD is effectively the same as average RFD, it is calculated at various time-intervals (e.g. 0-30, 0-50, 0-90, 0-100, 0-150, 0-200, and 0-250 milliseconds). This value simply represents a change in force divided by a change in time. It is calculated by dividing the force at the end of the time interval by the duration of the time interval. Just note that when calculating RFD, the time should be calculated in seconds, not milliseconds.

How to Calculate Time-interval RFD

Example – Calculating RFD with a 0-30 millisecond time-interval:

RFD [$N \cdot s^{-1}$] = Change in Force [N]/Change in Time [s]

RFD [$N \cdot s^{-1}$] = Force [N] at 30 milliseconds/0.03 second time-interval [s]

RFD [$N \cdot s^{-1}$] = 50N/0.03s

RFD [$N \cdot s^{-1}$] = 1,666

Table: Time-interval RFD calculations for the isometric mid-thigh clean pull.

Time (Ms)	Force (N)	Change in Force	Change in Time (s)	Change in Force/ Change in Time	RFD (N.s^{-1})
0-30	50	50	0.03	50/0.03	1,666
0-50	180	180	0.05	180/0.05	3,600
0-90	540	540	0.09	540/0.09	6,000
0-100	600	600	0.1	590/0.1	5,900
0-150	850	850	0.15	850/0.15	5,666
0-200	1,200	1,200	0.2	1190/0.2	5,950
0-250	1,400	1,400	0.25	1400/0.25	5,600

The strength and conditioning coach should select the time-intervals they wish to use based upon the nature of the exercise. For example, if the exercise has a fast-SSC movement (e.g. Sprinting – 80-90 milliseconds), then it may be suggested that time-intervals of ≤100 milliseconds may be most appropriate (e.g. 0-50, 0-90, and 0-100 milliseconds). Furthermore, the early time-intervals (<100ms) are often referred to as 'early phase' RFD, whilst >100s time-intervals are referred to as 'late phase' RFD.

Instantaneous RFD: This value is measured by using the maximal tangential slope between two adjacent data points. In other words, the data is recorded using 1-milliseconds time-intervals, and from this, the change in force is divided by the change in time at every 1-millisecond time interval. As this value of RFD is calculated every 1-millisecond, it provides a very precise measure of RFD.

Peak or Maximal RFD: This value of RFD is really as simple as it sounds, it is the largest amount of RFD produced during the movement. Most commonly, the value is identified by measuring the peak RFD during numerous sampling windows of 1, 2, 5, 10, 20, 30, and 50. For example, if the strength and conditioning coach selected a sampling window of 5 milliseconds, they would measure peak RFD every 5-milliseconds (e.g. 0-5, 5-10, and 10-15 milliseconds and so forth). They would then simply identify the largest RFD value out of those recorded – this value is then the peak RFD. Whilst all of these sampling windows have been reported as reliable measures of peak RFD, the 20-millisecond sampling window has been shown to be the most reliable. Table demonstrates how to identify peak RFD during an isometric performance.

Table: Peak RFD calculation using 50-millisecond sampling windows.

Time (Ms)	Force (N)	Change in Force (N)	Change in Time (s)	Change in Force/ Change in Time	R F - D(N.s^{-1})
0-50	180	180	0.05	180/0.05	3,600
50-100	600	420	0.05	420/0.05	8,400
100-150	850	250	0.05	250/0.05	5,000

150-200	1,200	350	0.05	350/0.05	7,000
200-250	1,400	200	0.05	200/0.05	4,000
Peak RFD					8,400
Time to Peak RFD (Ms)					100
Average RFD (peak force/time to peak force)					5,600

From this data, the coach is able to calculate the athlete's peak RFD, time to peak RFD, and average RFD. These variables are useful tools for comparing a group of athletes to identify who the best and worst individuals are at developing force quickly.

Time to Peak RFD: As displayed in table, this value of RFD is extremely straight-forward. It is a useful tool for measuring performance as it provides the coach with information on how quickly the athlete is able to achieve their maximal explosive strength (i.e. peak RFD). Decreasing an athlete's time to achieve peak RFD will allow them to produce higher forces in shorter periods of time, and therefore may increase their explosiveness and overall athletic performance.

Validity and Reliability

The RFD and its various measures (Average RFD, Time-Interval RFD, Peak RFD, and Time to Peak RFD) have all been shown to be a valid and reliable tool for assessing explosive strength. However, the most reliable measures for assessing RFD appears to be any of the time-interval sampling windows (i.e. 0-30, 0-50, 0-90, 0-100, 0-150, 0-200, and 0-250 milliseconds), and peak RFD using 20-millisecond windows (39). It is therefore recommended that these two variables should be preferable when measuring RFD.

Practical Application: How to improve the Rate of Force Development

Increasing the RFD whilst simultaneously reducing the time in which peak RFD occurs, will result in a left and upward shift in the force-time curve. This left and upward shift enables the athlete to produce greater forces in a shorted period of time, ultimately improving their explosiveness.

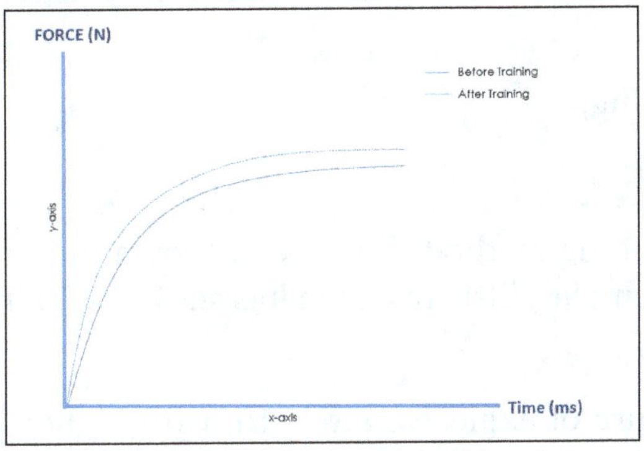

Shift in the Force-Time curve after a successful training programme.

It is often suggested that athletes must train at various sections along the force-time curve if improvements in RFD are to occur. By only training on one part of the force-time curve (e.g. maximum strength), it is likely that the athlete will only improve their performance at that section on the paradigm. For example, only training maximal strength may lead to improvements in force production, but it may also result in a reduction in the time to achieve that force.

As training programmes which combine strength and power training have been repeatedly shown to improve athletic performance more than strength or speed training alone, there is no surprise that most exercise professionals commonly use an all-rounded approach within their programming.

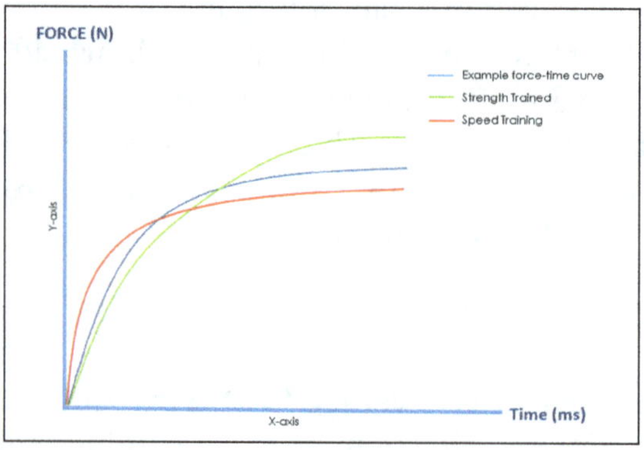

Force-time curve after training specific elements.

The following types of training have all shown to improve RFD:

- Resistance training,
- Ballistic training,
- Olympic weightlifting,
- Plyometric training,
- Balance training.

However, only those listed below have shown RFD improvements in trained or athletic subjects:

- Resistance training,
- Ballistic training.

So whilst numerous training methods have been shown to improve RFD in untrained and elderly males and females, little research has shown RFD improvements in trained or athletic subjects.

RFD is a reliable measure of explosive strength, with higher RFDs have been linked with better athletic performance. Improvements in RFD are likely to be the result of increases in muscle-tendon stiffness, enhanced muscle force production via changes in muscle fibre type (from type I to type IIA), and increases in neural drive. The most reliable values for measuring this component of performance appear to be calculating RFD at various time-intervals and peak RFD using 20-millisecond sampling windows. Though various methods of training have been shown to improve performance (resistance, ballistic, Olympic Weightlifting, plyometrics, and balance training), only resistance and ballistic training have been proven to increase RFD in trained and athletic populations.

Transfer of Strength and Power Training to Sports Performance

The ability to generate relatively high forces against large resistances (strength) and to produce a high work rate (power) is important for various sports. As such, resistance training has become an integral component of the physical preparation for enhancement of sports performance, and strength and conditioning training has become a specialization within sports training. A key issue for athletes and coaches at all levels is efficiency of training, that is, achieving the greatest gains in performance for a given amount of work effort. Therefore, the concept of maximizing the transfer of training to performance is paramount.

Transfer may be conceptually expressed as being a function of the following: gain in performance/gain in trained exercise (modified from Zatsiorsky). For example, using the data of Wilson 8 weeks of strength training with the squat exercise produced a 21% gain in the one-repetition-maximum (1RM) squat. This change was accompanied by an improvement in vertical-jump (VJ) performance of 21% and 40-m sprint performance of 2.3%. This example shows that training to improve leg strength as measured by a 1RM squat has excellent transference to VJ performance but considerably less to sprinting performance. Key issues involve determining the factors responsible for attaining high levels of transfer and whether appropriate training guidelines have been identified.

Central to the concept of transfer is the well-accepted training principle of specificity, which states that adaptations are specific to the nature of the training stress. If this principle is followed to the extreme, all training would simply mimic competition demands. Although such an approach may be expected to yield a good transfer to performance in the short term and in experienced athletes, it might also be expected to produce negative outcomes such as overtraining, muscle imbalances, increased injury risk, and boredom in the long term. If only specific training were used by athletes, many popular resistance-training modalities would never be used.

Approximately 60 years ago, coaches acknowledged that there was a role for general or nonspecific training to provide a "foundation" of fitness. More recently, general training has come to be thought valuable because it allows the development of a balanced neuromuscular system and serves as a base from which to train more specifically at later stages. Beginner athletes can achieve good transfer from general training, whereas experienced athletes attain specific adaptations. This suggests that the principle of specificity of training becomes more relevant according to the levels of training experience and performance.

Sprinting

Considerable research has indicated significant correlations between sprinting performance over various distances and a range of measures of strength and power. Significant relationships between strength and power and sprint performance imply that the muscle function assessed by strength and power tests has some commonality with performance. This might suggest that improvement in strength and power may lead to improvement in sprint performance, but because correlation does not indicate cause and effect, it is necessary to examine longitudinal studies involving resistance-training programs.

Sprint performance can be considered to contain 3 independent components: Acceleration, maximum speed, and speed maintenance. Statistical analysis of 100-m sprint running has confirmed this classification. Squats and jump squats (JS, loaded vertical jumps) are popular exercises for training strength and power, respectively, and have also been used in training studies. High-resistance weight training of the leg-extensor muscles is effective for improving maximum strength in a squat test, but this has not transferred to sprint speed. For example, Harris reported that 9 weeks of training with various squat and pulling exercises produced an approximately 10% gain in squat strength, but this was associated with no change in 30-m sprint performance. One study was able to demonstrate statistically significant gains in 40-m sprint performance after 8 weeks of squat training. To achieve a 2.2% gain in sprint performance, however, a 21% improvement in squat strength was required.

Although sprint performance may be more related to power than to strength, similar findings have been reported for power training. Training with either JS or plyometric exercise has been shown to produce significant gains in jump tests of leg power with small and nonsignificant changes in sprint performance. Experienced male sprinters who trained with various weight-training machines that involved hip and knee extensors and flexors were able to improve their 1RM squat by 12.4%. The corresponding improvements in acceleration and maximum speed, however, were only 4.3% and 1.9%, respectively. One study required subjects to perform JS with the load that yielded maximum power output over a 10-week period. The mean improvement in JS height using a 4-kg bar was 16.8%, but this was associated with only a 1.1% change in 30-m sprint time. In all of these studies, the power training consisted of exercises involving VJ performed bilaterally.

The poor transfer of power training could relate to a lack of movement specificity to sprinting, which involves unilateral contractions of the leg extensors resulting in total body movement in a horizontal direction. This suggestion is consistent with the findings of Rimmer and Sleivert, who reported that 8 weeks of plyometric training including some unilateral/horizontal exercises induced significant improvements (2.6%) in sprint time to 10 m. Furthermore, a 9-week sprint and plyometric program including both unilateral and horizontal exercises improved sprint performance to 10 m significantly more than sprinting alone, and, interestingly, the improved 10-m performance did carry over to 100-m performance. In these plyometric training studies, however, the benefits to short sprints did not extend to maximum speed.

The ability of some plyometric exercises to transfer to sprinting might partially reflect the contraction velocity specificity. Bounding exercises have been found to possess ground-contact times very similar to those of the acceleration phase of sprinting. In contrast, even low-resistance JS involve push-off times that are relatively long, such as >0.7 second. This point is worthy of elaboration. The rationale for using relatively light loads in resistance exercises is to produce a combination of contraction force and movement velocity that approximates maximum power output. Cronin conducted a study with nonresistance-trained females who performed bench-press throws with 60% of the predicted 1RM for 6 weeks. This load is considered "light" because in untrained women, 20 bench-press repetitions can be performed with this load. Bench-press throws with 60% of 1RM allowed a mean bar velocity of 0.4 m/s to be generated. When the same subjects executed a maximum-effort netball pass, the average ball speed generated was 11.4 m/s. In this example, the "light load/high speed" resistance exercise produced a movement speed representing only 3.5% of the speed attained in the netball pass. This shortcoming highlights the difficulty of achieving sport-specific movement velocities with many resistance-training exercises.

Alternatives to exercises such as JS or bench-press throws with barbells are plyometric exercise (discussed above) and the performance of the sport skill with added load. An example of the latter is sprinting while pulling a loaded sled. A study that compared unresisted and sled-resisted sprinting indicated that a sled load of 12.5% of body mass produced a running velocity that was 90% of the unresisted velocity over 15 m. The authors concluded that this load would be suitable for training because it produced minimal disruption to sprint mechanics but still provided the necessary overload. Furthermore, it appears that achieving movement and velocity specificity is easier with this mode of resistance training. A recent study evaluated the effects of sled sprint training with a 5-kg load (about 7% of body mass) on sprint performance. Eight repetitions of 20- to 50-m sprints performed over an 8-week period produced a significant 2.0% gain in running velocity over the first 20 m, but no improvement in maximum speed was attained. These findings are expected because sprinting mechanics using a sled are more similar to the acceleration phase (eg, more forward lean) than the maximum-speed phase of sprinting.

Resisted sports movements such as sled sprinting could potentially hinder sports performance if the skill is dramatically changed. This concern is probably unfounded for

2 reasons. First, the greater the additional load used in sled sprinting, the greater the modification to the unresisted sport skill. Therefore, the use of a relatively light load, such as the 12.5% of body mass recommended by Lockie et al, should ensure minimal alteration of the correct mechanics. Second, the volume of this type of resistance training would be far less than the quantity of unresisted sprint training, which would further minimize any expected biomechanical disruption over time. Nevertheless, more longitudinal research concerning the potential benefits of many resisted-sprinting methods is needed.

Physiological basis of Transfer

Strength and power production in sport are influenced by a range of neuromuscular factors. In simple terms, muscle performance is determined by a combination of muscle cross-sectional area and the extent to which the muscle mass is activated, that is, neural factors. Sprinting is influenced by neuromuscular function, and, because of its complexity, many different muscles must be activated at the appropriate times and intensities to maximize speed.

Because muscle cross-sectional area is related to voluntary strength, hypertrophy training methods potentially increase force and power output in a sports movement. With regard to enhancing sports performance, an important consideration with hypertrophy training is the concept of optimum muscle and total body mass. Gains in muscle size are associated with gains in body mass, and such changes may or may not enhance sports performance, depending on the needs of the individual. For example, hypertrophy methods might be appropriate for a shot-putter seeking gains in absolute strength and power, but they could reduce the power:weight ratio of a high jumper and therefore inhibit high-jump performance.

According to Carroll, the physiological adaptations associated with resistance training can potentially produce either positive or negative transfer to sports performance. Negative transfer could occur if there is increased coactivation of antagonist muscles because this would produce force that opposes the intended movement direction. For example, Baratta et al showed that knee-flexion training produced greater knee-flexion activation during a knee-extension strength test. This observation indicates that the training of the hamstrings caused this muscle group to produce greater antagonistic coactivation during the knee-extension task. Positive transfer can occur if resistance training reinforces the optimum muscle-activation patterns that are required in the execution of the sport skill. This could be achieved by either increased excitatory neural activation of muscles that contribute to skillful performance and by inhibition of muscles that can degrade performance. Apart from decreased cocontraction of antagonists, transfer might be enhanced by improved interaction between synergists. Generally, the improved coordination of muscles involved in a sports movement has been termed intermuscular coordina-tion and is considered important for sprint performance.

The importance of intermuscular coordination for achieving transfer from training to athletic performance is demonstrated by 2 studies involving different methodologies. In the first study, Bobbert and Van Soest used a computer simulation of VJ performance from input of force produced over time by 6 lower extremity muscles. First, the model was optimized to maximize jump height using parameters similar to those recorded from well-trained volleyball players. When only muscle force was increased to simulate increased muscle strength, it was found that jump height decreased. For example, a 20% increase in knee-extensor force in isolation produced a 9-cm decrease in jump height. When the model was reoptimized using this enhanced muscle force, jump height was improved by 3 cm beyond the original performance. This finding indicates that jump performance could be impaired by altered intermuscular coordination, despite increased force output from individual muscles. The authors concluded that to improve jumping performance, a precise tuning of the control of muscle properties must be achieved.

The second study required subjects to perform 3 sets of 10 repetitions of an isokinetic knee-extension and -flexion exercise at 100°/s for 6 weeks. After 6 weeks of training each leg unilaterally, the mean gain in quadriceps and hamstrings isokinetic strength assessed at the training velocity was between 7% and 11.8% and was statistically significant for the quadriceps. Improvements in standing long-jump performance were more modest (2.3%) and not significant, despite the fact that this activity significantly involves the quadriceps and hamstring muscles. Because the subjects in this study did not practice jumping during the training period, it could be speculated that the intermuscular coordination was not optimal and may have limited the transfer from the training. The relatively poor transfer might also be explained by a violation of the specificity principle. Sale and MacDougall suggested that training should be specific in terms of movement pattern, contraction velocity, contraction type, and contraction force. The training exercise differed from the standing long jump with regard to all of these factors.

Intermuscular coordination refers to the interaction between muscles that control a movement, but neural adaptations confined to a single muscle might also explain performance enhancement from training and have thus been termed intramuscular coordination. These include such factors as increased motor-unit recruitment, firing rates, and synchronization, as well as reflex potentiation and decreased inhibition from eccentric loads during stretch–shorten cycle contractions to optimize musculotendinous stiffness.

Although the measurement of these individual mechanisms is complex, changes in neural activation as recorded by surface electromyography (EMG) have been clearly demonstrated in resistance-training studies. Yet despite significant gains in the neural activation of individual muscles, transfer to specific sports movements can be limited. For example, McBride reported that subjects who trained for 8 weeks with JS using 80% of their 1RM squat achieved an increase of greater than 60% in the average EMG output of the vastus lateralis while performing JS. This was accompanied by a smaller 10% gain (statistically significant) in peak power output while jumping and no improvement in jump height or sprinting performance. This finding indicates that intramuscular coordination factors might be relatively less influential than intermuscular factors and reinforces the importance of movement-pattern specificity for transfer to jumping and sprinting performance.

Role of General Resistance Training

The specificity of resistance training for transfer to sports performance has been highlighted. Therefore, what is the role, if any, for general or nonspecific resistance training? First, general strength training has been shown to transfer to performance in skills such as VJ5 and baseball-throwing velocity. For example, strength training using bench-press and pull-over exercises for 8 weeks produced a 22.8% gain in 6RM strength, and this was accompanied by a significant improvement (4.1%) of baseball-throwing velocity. The subjects in this study had a mean age of 18.6 years and no previous experience in resistance training. It is not clear whether similar gains could occur from general strength training in highly strength-trained baseball players.

Another proposed benefit of general strength training is a reduction in the risk of sports injuries such as damage to soft tissues. As such, a significant portion of an athlete's time in physical preparation might be devoted to this goal. For example, eccentric strength training for the hamstrings has been recommended for the prevention and rehabilitation from hamstring strains and has been shown to be effective for injury reduction using a prospective randomized controlled research design. General strength training of the muscles of the lower extremity has also been shown to be just as effective or more effective46 than balance training for enhancing balance and proprioception. Because balance capabilities have been linked to sports-injury risk, strength training might have a prophylactic benefit.

The development of core stability has also become a focus of many strength and conditioning programs, especially in junior athletes.48 Core stability is thought to be important for sprint-running efficiency. Research using a prospective design50 indicated that hip-abduction and external-rotation strength were significantly lower in athletes who were subsequently injured during a season and led the authors to conclude that core stability has an important role in injury prevention. However, 6 weeks of corestability training in recreational athletes has been shown to enhance measures of core stability, without significant transfer to running economy or performance.

Although a strong connection between core-stability training and injury prevention is yet to be established by researchers, 2 key issues for strength and conditioning professionals have emerged. The first is determining the proportion of the program devoted to injury prevention and general training compared with specific training designed to maximize transfer to sports performance directly. The second is the appropriate ways in which to develop core stability, as there is a large range of exercise possibilities.

General strength training might be beneficial for athletes because of the potential to enhance the force-generating capabilities of muscle, increase total body mass, reduce the risk of sports injuries, and improve core stability. However, direct transfer to improve sports performance might be limited by such training in experienced athletes. Although nonspecific resistance training can induce neural adaptations and increase the power production of individual muscles, it appears that to maximize transfer to specific sports skills, training should be as specific as possible, especially with regard to movement pattern and contraction velocity. This type of training can be expected to enhance intermuscular coordination and ensure that muscles are "tuned" to any newly acquired force-generating capacity. Adding a load to a sports movement would seem to be a suitable strategy to achieve this specificity, although the amount and direction of added resistance would need to be considered.

Ultimately, a combination of general and specific resistance-training methods can be recommended to develop all the neuromuscular factors contributing to sports skills requiring strength and power. The way in which these methods are integrated over time is an issue of periodization that must be considered and is likely to depend on the needs and developmental level of the individual athlete. A developing athlete might be advised to emphasize core stability, muscle hypertrophy (if increased body mass is advantageous), and intramuscular coordination. Provided a solid foundation has been developed, a highly resistance-trained athlete might be expected to benefit more from training intermuscular coordination.

It may be useful to think of training an athlete to improve sprinting performance by using an analogy of a competitive sports car. General training may include hypertrophy to increase the force-generation capacities of important muscles, as well as strengthening core muscles. The second training strategy is to develop the "neural activation capacity" of the relevant muscles. Although these combined approaches might build a powerful athlete, maximization of transfer to sports performance requires the "conversion" of powerful muscles to a coordinated sports skill.

Table: Strategies for developing power in a sprinter based on neuromuscular factors using an analogy of a race car.

Race-car performance	Sprinting performance	Example of neuromuscular factors	Training methods
↑ engine capacity	↑ muscle crosssectional area	↑ muscle crosssectional area	Hypertrophy with squats

↑ engine power output, eg, optimum timing of all cylinders	↑ intramuscular coordination of involved muscles	↑ motor-unit recruitment, fi ring rates, synchronization, refl ex potentiation	Jump squats with load that maximizes power output
↑ conversion of power from engine to road, eg, effective transmission	↑ intermuscular coordination	↑ activation of synergists, ↓ cocontraction of antagonists	Resisted sprints, unilateral/horizontal plyometrics, eg, speed bounding

Stability Principles and Balance in Sports

Stability principles give athletes rules about holding positions and staying on balance when running. They guide training for improving firmness of positions both for static balance and dynamic balance.

An athlete's center of gravity is the exact middle of the body around which it can rotate freely in any direction and where the weight balanced on all opposite sides. It exists at a point along the midline of the body at about 55% of the athlete's height.

Stability Principles

1. To maintain balance when still, the athlete's center of gravity must remain over the base of support. For example, beginning a free weight lifting movement, such as the squat, requires the lifter to hold a standing position.

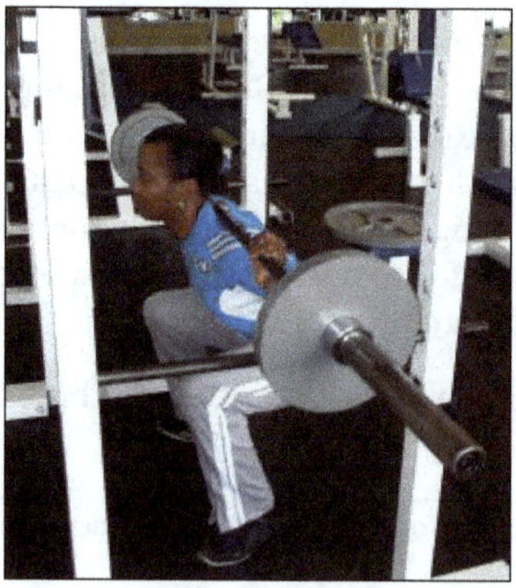

2. To regain balance when lost, an athlete can enlarge the base of support and reposition the center of gravity over it. Example: Placing the feet wider to prevent falling after being pushed helps recover balance.

3. When lifting or carrying an object, shift the body weight in order to maintain balance. Example: Lean in the opposite direction when carrying a heavy equipment bag.

4. For greatest stability in all directions, the center of gravity should be over the center of the base of support. Example: Holding a handstand requires the hips to remain toward the center of the base formed by the hands.

5. An athlete can become more stable by lowering the center of gravity. Example: A shotput followthrough involves bending the knees to prevent fouling.

6. The greater the friction between the supporting surface and the athlete's body, the greater the ability to maintain balance. Example: Wearing shoes that prevent excessive sliding on a playing surface.

7. Shifting the center of gravity toward an approaching force increases an athlete's ability to maintain balance. Example: A football lineman shifts weight toward the opposing line prior to the snap.

8. An opponent can be forced to lose balance if pushed or pulled in the direction where the center of gravity is closest to the edge of the base of support. Example: Boxers can lose balance when weight is shifted back on the heels.

9. For positions of readiness, the shorter the distance the center of gravity must move to clear the base of support, the more rapidly the body can be put in motion in that direction. Example: Sprinters in the "set" position shift their weight in the direction of the race.

A successful athlete does not always need to be stable, though in general, athletes need to maintain balance. As athletes become more and more unbalanced, they lose control and find it more difficult to complete a desired task.

In many sports, it is the strategy of the opponent to disrupt the balance of the competitor, leaving the competitor more vulnerable to mistakes. For instance, when a defender jumps and puts a hand in the air while the player on offense is trying to shoot, the person shooting will do everything possible to avoid being rejected. Great players, such as Michael Jordan, are experts at maintaining balance in the absence of stability. Arms and legs fly everywhere, but still the movement seems smooth because of their ability to maintain balance while adjusting the shot in mid-air. Less talented players will attempt to adjust, but because they are unable to maintain balance, the shot comes off awkwardly, usually missing the mark by a good amount.

Consequently, if a player were trying to lose a defender as he/she drives towards the basket, the objective would be to upend the stability of the foe. It is much more difficult to defend with flailing arms than by keeping the body between the offensive player and the basket. A player could easily hook around an outstretched arm, as long as the basketball is protected.

However, if the offensive player is unable to move around a defender, the player might be forced to take a shot further away from the basket than desired. Depending on how quickly the defender reacts, the player on offense might also be forced to take a shot while off balance. It is therefore imperative that a good defender keep his/her legs underneath him/her, the chest a little forward and the arms outstretched in order to maintain stability and ease of movement.

Stability is also necessary for a good free-throw shooter. The idea when shooting a free-throw is to be able to repeat and to produce the power needed to shoot the ball with the legs and core of the body. This allows the arms to be free and enables the shooter to propel the ball up instead of out. If the greater mass of the body is not maintained between the feet while shooting, the player must then rely on the strength of the arms to loft the ball, usually resulting in a "line-drive" shot.

A soccer goalie has similar objectives to the basketball defender. The goalie must always be in a "ready" stance, meaning ready to move in any direction quickly. It is the stable goalie who can stay between the ball and the goal. An offensive player may try to fake the goalie into moving in one direction, and then kick it in the other direction. This will cause the lower body of the goalie to move out from under the upper body, forcing him/her to try and block the ball with just a hand.

Stability is of the utmost importance to offensive linemen in football. Their main goal is to protect the quarterback, or whoever has the ball, by blocking the defenders. Offensive linemen are usually large in stature because it is easier to maintain stability when being pushed by the defense. Typically, their balance is not very good, because once they start to fall, they fall hard and fast, with little time for recovery of balance.

Offensive linemen work hard on moving the feet quickly so as to stay in front of their defender, staying in a "ready" rather than upright position and keeping their hands in front of them. All of these elements improve stability and make it more difficult for the defender to get around them.

Running backs rely heavily on balance to charge and dance their way to the end zone, as do wide receivers. Many of the best wide receivers are good because they can make catches while being pushed, shoved, and even tripped. The receivers are often running full bore, and unless the ball is perfectly thrown, they have to adjust to catch the ball. As their mass is moving in one direction at full speed, slowing down or stopping becomes very tricky. A reception called a "circus catch" is named so because the usually wiry receiver has to manipulate his/her body and make an incredible catch either by reaching high into the air, diving, or catching a tipped ball. All of these circumstances warrant a high degree of bodily control or ability to balance.

The position of shortstop in baseball calls for a player who is agile, athletic, and able to make strong throws from odd positions. The basic motion of throwing a baseball will show the player stepping towards the intended target, widening the stance, and lowering the center of gravity, allowing the arm to wind up behind the throwing shoulder and then turning the chest towards and then left (if right handed) of the target, releasing the ball.

A ground ball that is hit directly at a fielder will allow the player to follow the basic motion of throwing. Unfortunately, often the ball is not fielded directly in front of the body. One of the toughest throws for any right-handed player is to be fielding the ball away from first base. As the player's momentum carries him/her to the right, the ball must be propelled across the body and to the left. A player who has poor balance will usually throw the ball away. The momentum takes over and the body is unable to balance itself while the throw is being made.

Similarly, if the player has poor stability before the ball is hit (perhaps from standing too upright with the weight heading towards the heels) it will cause the fielder time in getting to the ball because he/she must stabilize himself first. Another result could be that the fielder does catch the ball, but in an unbalanced position.

Trying to keep the body stable while making a swing from a static position seems as though it should be easy. Often in golf, a student will be told to swing as hard as possible while in balance. It is not as easy as it looks.

A golfer must maintain a posture that allows the center of gravity to be towards the middle of the body as he/she bends forward with an implement in hand which measures anywhere from 35 to 48 inches. Consequently, he/she must hold this posture to swings the implement (club) while trying to create momentum to propel a golf ball up to 300+ yards.

For instance, if the weight, or center of gravity, is positioned too far towards the toes in order to maintain balance during the swing, the golfer will appear to rock back and then forward. If the body did not compensate, the golfer would fall forward as he/she swung the club back.

From the frontal position, the vertical line of balance does not dissect the spine and head. On a right-handed golfer, the upper spine is tilted slightly to the right. There is a little more weight distributed to the right side, then, at address. This is caused by the right hand being lower on the club than the left. If at any time before impact there is a larger amount of mass in front of the line as opposed to behind, it unfavorably changes how the club comes down to the ball.

There is also a saying in golf instruction that a player should swing between the feet. This is directly related to stability, as the feet are the foundation of the body mass. If the stance is too narrow, as the golfer swings the mass will sway from one side to the other. The weight will be forced outside the right ankle on the way back and from there, many things could happen. The center of gravity could be too high, causing it to move back and forth due to the momentum of the swinging club. If the stance is too wide for that particular player, the center of gravity could lower so much that it inhibits a turning motion and instead fosters a back and forth swaying motion.

Good balance is imperative in movements in which the player is being forced in different directions. Stability is very important to those who wish to maintain a consistent center of gravity. An athlete can be unstable, but in balance. A wide receiver's center of gravity will change as he/she manipulates his/her body to catch a ball. As long as the wide receiver maintains control of his/her body, or balance, it will be possible to attempt the catch.

The offensive lineman is more concerned with stability. Although on the offensive team, the lineman is defending the quarterback and running backs, and knows he/she will be pushed. Therefore the lineman lowers his/her center of gravity and keeps his/her feet under him/her to stay stable.

A baseball player fielding a ground ball and throwing it to first must foremost be stable in order to move efficiently to the ball. However, often the sharpness of the hit causes the center of gravity to change rapidly as he/she lunges or dives toward the ball. It is then that balance must be maintained in order to not only catch the ball, but to quickly recover so that an accurate throw can ensue.

Defensive players typically are concerned with stability in the sports of basketball and soccer. Hockey could be added to this group as well, but stability is automatically compromised because the lack of friction.

Basketball defenders must move their feet quickly and keep their upper bodies on top of the lower body in order to move with the man who has the ball. If this is done, it will allow the defender's center of gravity to remain lower and more consistent. This slows down the offensive players and hopefully forces them to adjust their shots.

A soccer goalie is similar in that the objective is to keep his/her feet below his/her mass to project more of a presence within the goal, making it easier to attempt to block the ball with the body and arms rather than just the hands.

When addressing the golf ball, golfers concentrate on a good posture, fostering more stability. Once the club is swung into motion, a golfer will adjust for balance if the stability, or center of gravity, is not towards the middle of the body.

Balance is something that is affected by many factors. How a person perceives, thinks, and reacts about the environment around him/her controls it. Those who are successful at good balance appear fluid and athletic. Those who are not look awkward and jerky.

Stability is an objective for those who wish to maintain control of the mass of the body while moving or being moved. It can be the basis of balance because if the center of gravity is being shifted, it causes the athlete to try and regain balance.

Balance and stability work together to assist an athlete in making efficient movements. Although the definitions are not the same, they are intertwined in that they do affect one another. It is very difficult to talk about one and not the other.

Kinetic Energy

Kinetic energy is the energy an object has because of its motion. It is also defined as the amount of energy gained by an object from the state of rest to motion. The object maintains this kinetic energy unless its speed changes. If the speed of this object changes from the state of motion to rest, then same amount of kinetic energy is lose by the object.

All moving objects have kinetic energy. For example, the earth revolving around the sun, electrons orbiting the nucleus of an atom, birds flying in the sky, trains moving on tracks, cars moving on road have kinetic energy. If the kinetic energy does not exist, everything around us will be motionless. All objects would be unable to move. The entire universe would be cold because heat is also a form of kinetic energy.

The kinetic energy of an object is mathematically written as:

$$K = \frac{1}{2} mv^2$$

where,

K = Kinetic energy,

m = mass of an object,

v = velocity of an object.

The kinetic energy of an object depends on its mass and velocity. For a given velocity, the kinetic energy of an object is directly proportional to its mass. Similarly, for a given mass, the kinetic energy of an object is directly proportional to its velocity.

Kinetic energy is a scalar quantity; it has only magnitude and does not have any direction. Kinetic energy is measured in joules.

The concept of kinetic energy can be easily understood by a simple example that demonstrates how kinetic energy is converted in to another form of energy. For example, a sports person uses chemical energy provided by food to run to a chosen speed. Here, the chemical energy in the sports person has been converted in to kinetic energy. But, the process is not completely efficient because some amount of chemical energy is converted in to heat energy. During constant motion sports person maintains this kinetic energy. However, if he slows down and comes to rest position, then he loses the same amount of kinetic energy.

Kinetic energy can also be passed from one object to other. For example, in the game of billiards, the player supplies kinetic energy to the cue ball by striking it with the cue stick. The cue ball maintains this kinetic energy unless its speed changes. If this cue ball collides with another cue ball, then it supplies kinetic energy to that ball by losing its kinetic energy. The ball with which it collided will start moving due to gaining of kinetic energy.

Relation between Work and Energy

Work W performed by external forces that are acting on a body is the cause of the change of energy ΔE of the body:

$$W = \Delta E$$

Let us have a look at a shot-putter, for example. He used a force of 1206 N to displace the shot by 0.5 m in the direction of the throw. The force used was constant. We will neglect vertical displacement of the shot and thus also its potential energy. Let us imagine that all work was used up to change the kinetic energy of the shot. If we know that the work of 603 J was performed, then the change of the kinetic energy of the shot in the place of throw was 603 J. What was the velocity vodhod of the shot weighing 7.26 kg at the moment of the throw?

$$W = \Delta E$$

$$(630 \text{ J}) = \frac{1}{2}(7,26 \text{ kg})\, v_{\text{odhod}}^2$$

$$v_{\text{odhod}} = \sqrt{\frac{2(603 \text{ J})}{7,26 \text{ kg}}}$$

$$v_{\text{odhod}} = 12,88 \text{ m/ s}$$

The initial velocity of the shot at the moment of the throw was 12,88 m/s, as it follows from the relation between work and the change of kinetic energy. The increase in the mechanical energy of the shot equals only the increase in its kinetic energy, because we decided to neglect its potential energy.

Increasing Energy by Performing Work

In sport and physical exercise we often need to maximize kinetic energy of a given body. In order to maximize kinetic energy of human body or sport equipment we must exert the greatest possible force along the longest possible distance.

This way we can make us of the knowledge of the relation between energy and work to improve our technique in certain sports, especially in athletics. From the relation between impulse of force and momentum we know that for better technique and thus for increasing the velocity of a projectile we need to use greatest possible force for longest possible time. According to the relation between work and energy the velocity is maximized by the greatest possible force acting along the longest possible distance.

For example shot-putters must throw the shot from a shot-put circle according to the rules, from which they must not step out. Dimensions of the shot-put circle limit the shot-putters' possibility to perform work because they can exert force only along a limited distance. Shot-putters therefore often start their throw by standing on one foot, bent forward over the edge of the shot-put circle, with their back towards the direction of the throw, to maximize the distance along which their force will act on the shot and thus to also maximize the initial velocity of the shot at the moment of the throw. The longer distance along which the force acts on the shot and the ability to use larger muscle groups thus leads to longer throws and better results.

By performing work we can increase not only kinetic but also potential energy of a body.

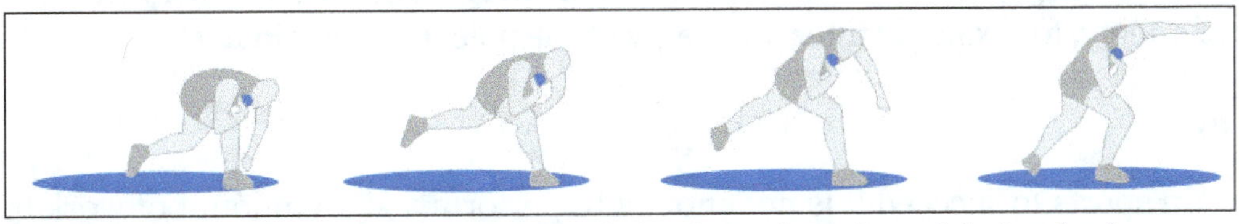

Initial phases of shot put allowing to maximize the work performed during the throw.

Decreasing Energy by Performing Work

The relation between energy and work can also be used to explain techniques of absorbing energy of a body to prevent potential injuries of athletes. This happens mostly in catching projectiles, landing, etc. when negative work is performed. Human muscles also perform negative work when our body lands on the ground. Energy of a human body during landing is simply given and forces caused by it can lead to injuries if we don't use the correct landing technique. During landing it is important to maximize the distance along which the projectile is decelerating. By making stopping distance longer we make impact forces smaller. We must realize, however, that prolonging the stopping distance by bending our knees deeply, for example, does not necessary lead to smaller reaction forces in specific joints. The resultant reaction force acting on the floor is smaller but for example in the knee the moment of force can even increase in comparison with landing by bending our knees less and then moving backward.

To decrease impact forces and increase stopping distance we also use various materials: Sand (long jump), water (diving), running shoes, boxing gloves, etc.

Law of Conservation of Mechanical Energy

If no work is performed on a body, it follows: Change of kinetic energy + change of potential energy + change of elastic energy = 0:

$$\Delta E_k + \Delta E_p + \Delta E_D = 0$$

$$\Delta\left(E_k + E_p + E_D\right) = 0$$

Total mechanical energy of a body is constant unless external forces act on it (other than gravitational force).

$$E_k + E_p + E_D = \text{Konst}.$$

This law can be used in studying the motion of projectiles. For example if we assume that a pole vaulter does not perform any work after taking off, his total mechanical energy at the beginning of the vault is equal to his kinetic energy at the end of his run-up. This kinetic energy is transformed into deformation energy of the pole and subsequently into the increase in potential energy of the athlete. In other words, the faster the pole vaulter runs and the better his pole is able to transform kinetic energy into potential energy through deformation energy, the higher he jumps. Part of energy is of course transformed in other types of energy, for example internal energy of the pole, resulting in heat.

Power

In certain sports to succeed it is not enough to perform a great amount of work but we must perform a great amount of work in the shortest possible time. In mechanics such ability is described by the quantity called power.

Average power describes the amount of work performed during a period of time. Mathematically this can be expressed as:

$$P = \frac{W}{t},$$

where P is power (W), W is work (J) a t is time period.

Instantaneous power is work performed over time period that is approaching zero.

Power Measures Speed with which Work is Performed

Power can also be defined as product of average force and average velocity of displacement of a body in the direction of that force:

$$P = \boldsymbol{F}\boldsymbol{v} = F_t v,$$

where P is average power (J), F is average force (N), F_t is the magnitude of the component of the average force in the direction of the body's displacement (N), v is the magnitude of the average velocity of the body's displacement in the direction of the average force (m/s), and v is the velocity of displacement (m/s).

Is it a good idea to swish arms when jumping up? What is the optimum gear ratio for cycling as fast as possible under the given conditions? What is the optimum length of step to walk as fast as possible under the given conditions? To answer these complicated questions it will help us to know the concept of power and also to know certain qualities of muscles.

In complex human motions the maximum output mechanical power is reached with approximately 50 % of maximum force and velocity of a given athlete. That could mean that the best gear ratio in cycling is not the top, neither the bottom, but somewhere between the both extremes. The optimum length of step in running is not the longest, neither the shortest but somewhere in between. The best choice of gear ratio, length of step, etc. is the one that allows your muscles to contract with optimum speed and optimum force, which results in maximum mechanical muscle power. In complex motor tasks the resulting power is influenced not only by qualities of individual muscles but also by muscle coordination.

Let us have a look again at weightlifting, specifically at the events of "clean and jerk" and "snatch". The force with which the weightlifter acts on the barbell and the velocity of his motion indicates enormous muscle power (about 3.200 W) but only for a very short time. If the time of motion were longer, would he still be able to produce such enormous power? Duration of physical activity substantially influences the ability to produce muscle power. Sprinters are able to maintain power for a relatively short period of time (0-60 s). Power outputs of runners at medium distances are markedly lower than that of sprinters because the duration of their motor activity is increased from one to seven minutes. Marathon runners produce even lower power output because they run for two to four hours. Human metabolic system influences the ability of athletes to produce power.

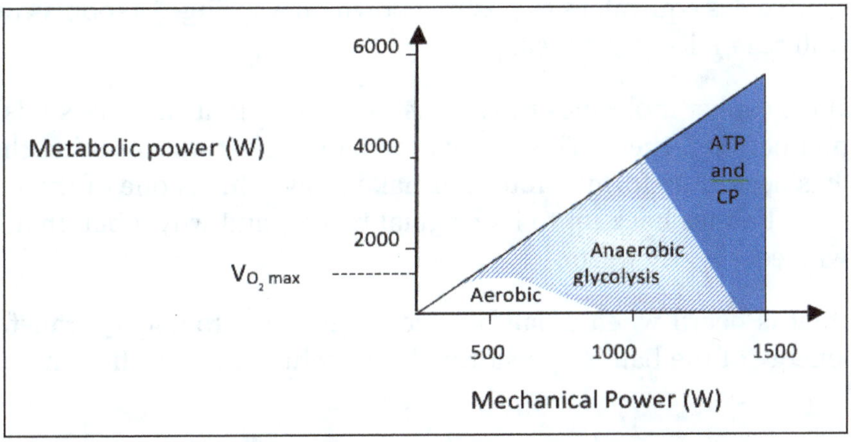

The relation between metabolic and mechanical power, and sources of energy (aerobic metabolism, anaerobic glycolysis, and high-energy phosphates).

Potential Energy

Potential Energy is the energy that can be stored in order to do work at a later time. For example, if a ball is lifted off the ground, it has potential energy. Gravity is an example of potential energy (called "gravitational potential").

Potential energy is the energy stored in an object. In other words, it is the capacity to do work at a later time. For example, if you lift a ball off the ground, it has the potential to fall. The higher the ball is off the ground, the more potential energy it has. As the ball falls to the ground, its potential energy decreases.

Kinetic energy is the energy an object has when it is in motion. The faster the object travels, the more kinetic energy it has.

When a ball is held in the air, it is not moving, and has no kinetic energy; but it does have a lot of potential energy. As the ball falls to the ground, the kinetic energy increases as the speed of the ball increases, but the potential energy decreases.

When a player sets the ball or makes a pass, the ball is propelled through the air in an arched trajectory. The ball is said to possess kinetic energy because it is in motion. However, whenever the ball is thrown in the air either straight up, or following an arched trajectory, there is a very brief moment just after the ball stops travelling upwards—but before it starts falling back to the ground—when the ball possesses very little vertical kinetic energy, but a lot of potential energy.

When the ball is held two metres above the ground, it does not have any kinetic energy (it is not moving), but it does have potential energy (stored energy). When the ball is let go, the potential energy is transformed into kinetic energy. When the ball hits the ground, it gets slightly squished and deformed. It thus acquires another form of potential energy, called elastic potential energy, as the rubber from the ball tries to regain its original shape. This is equivalent to pushing down on a spring. As soon as the spring is released, it will regain its original shape.

The fact that the rubber molecules rub against one another during this squishing phase causes friction between them. This causes the ball to heat up, meaning that some of the energy has been transformed into thermal energy. This is one of the reasons why the ball will not bounce back up to its original height, and why a ball that is bounced frequently will feel slightly warm.

The sound that is heard when a ball bounces is also due to energy transformation—the kinetic energy of the ball is transformed into sound energy when the ball hits the ground.

Impulse and Momentum

From Newton's Second Law of Motion indirectly follows also the relation between the duration of force and the change to motion of a human body or any object. This relation can be described with the help of two quantities: impulse of force and momentum. Impulse of force is the product of the resultant force ΣF and the duration of this force Δt, if the force is constant. Impulse of force is the cause of changes to motion and therefore changes to momentum. Mathematically this can be expressed as:

$$\sum \boldsymbol{F} \Delta t = m\,(\boldsymbol{v}_{\text{final}} - \boldsymbol{v}_{\text{initial}})$$

where m is the mass of the moving body, v_{final} is the velocity at the end of the time interval in question, $v_{initial}$ is the velocity at the beginning of the time interval in question.

The expression $m(v_{final} - v_{initial})$ describes the change to momentum Δp and the expression $\Sigma F \Delta t$ describes the impulse of force I.

To change momentum of a body we need to change its velocity or its mass. In sport and physical exercise there are mostly no changes in the mass of a human body, therefore a change to momentum is caused almost exclusively by changes to velocity.

Resultant external force acting on a human body for certain time causes changes to its momentum.

To cause greater change to momentum we have to either use greater force for the same period of time, or the same force for a longer period of time.

Using Impulse of Force to Increase Momentum in Sport

In many sports the elementary motor task is to change as much as possible the velocity of human body, its parts, or of an object. In throwing, kicking, tossing, and jumping the projectiles at the beginning of their motion have zero velocity. When fulfilling a motor task, for example throwing javelin, we are trying to give the javelin at the end of our motion the greatest possible velocity. We are therefore trying to increase the momentum of the javelin. The same follows for certain strokes in tennis, boxing and other sports. The important thing is that to change momentum we have to either use greater force or increase the duration of the same force.

The greater the impulse of force, the greater the change to momentum of a body (projectile, human body, tennis racket, ball, etc).

When throwing light objects, the technique used (duration of force) is much more important for the longest possible throw than the magnitude of the force. When throwing heavy objects, the magnitude of the force is more important. Shot-putters are usually stronger and bigger than javelin throwers. Their preparation is focused on enhancing their ability to exert great force (ΣF in the impulse of force). Top javelin throwers do not have the same maximum strength as shot-putters but they are successful because their technique maximizes the duration of the force they exert (Δt in the impulse of force).

Using Impulse of Force to Decrease Momentum in Sport

Certain sport activities, on the other hand, necessitate decreasing a high initial velocity of a human body (or an object) to zero velocity. In other words we need to decrease momentum of given bodies. As examples we can easily imagine all kinds of landing, catching of balls, pucks, etc.

For example pole vaulters cannot land on their feet, due to the technique they use, but they land on their backs. Landing on the hard ground means a very short time of deceleration of human body, so the forces acting on human body in such a situation would be massive and devastating. Landing pads are made of soft and floppy material which prolongs the time of breaking the fall. The impulse of force is the same as in landing on the ground but its magnitude is decided rather by the duration of landing than by the magnitude of the force. Gymnasts also do not land on the ground but on specially designed soft and flexible pads that prolong the time of breaking the fall to decrease impact forces acting on gymnasts.

Boxing gloves, catching glove of an ice hockey goal keeper, running shoes, and all kinds of other sporting equipment with the task of reducing substantial forces generated in contact with other bodies are based on the same principles.

Centre of Percussion

The center of percussion is the impact location which produces no reaction force at the pivot. It is only by coincidence that the COP is often located near the so-called "sweet spot" of the bat. While early bat performance tests prescribed impacts at the COP, modern methods do not use the COP.

The center of percussion (or COP) of a bat is the impact location that produces no reaction force at the pivot point. It may be distinguished from the balance point with a simple test (a kick). If a bat placed on the floor is kicked at its balance point, it will move forward, but not rotate in the plane of the floor (although it may roll about its long axis). If the same bat (still on the floor) is kicked at its COP, it will tend to rotate about the pivot point conjugate to the impact location. In bat testing, the pivot point from which the COP is defined, is usually 6 inches from the knob. (The pivot point, however, may be defined at any location of interest along the length of the bat).

In physics or dynamics courses a bat impact is sometimes incorrectly cited as an example to explain the COP. It is argued that when a ball strikes the COP, the hands feel no reaction force, providing the so called "sweet spot." The sting a player feels in the hands from a poorly hit ball is due to bat vibration, however, not a reaction force. It is only a coincidence that the COP of a bat is often close to the location that minimizes bat vibration. In spite of experimental and theoretical evidence supporting the independence of the COP and sweet spot, some maintain its significance. ASTM F1890, for instance, measures bat performance at the COP which is reported as BPF. The COP, relative to the pivot point, is found from,

$$COP = g\left(\frac{t}{2\pi}\right)^2$$

where t is the average period (in seconds) of the bat swinging freely about its pivot point, and g is the gravitational constant (386 in/s2). A detailed method describing how the COP is measured can be found in ASTM F2398. The COP will typically lie between 21 and 22 inches from the pivot point of a 34 inch long bat.

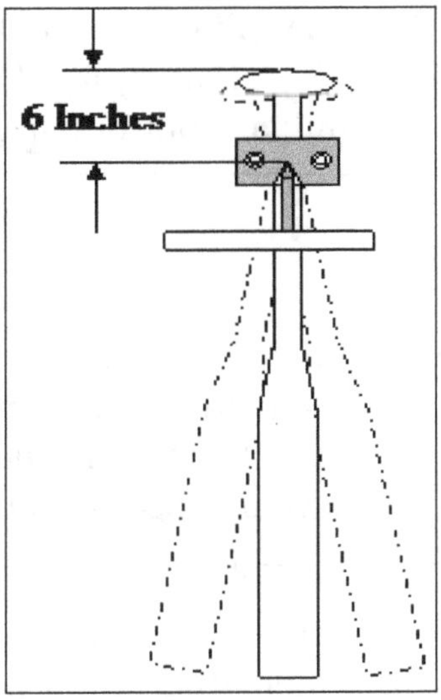

Schematic of bat swinging freely about its pivot point.

Angular Kinematics

Angular kinematics follows many of the conventions as linear kinematics. However, angular kinematics often involves several aspects of physical laws occurring simultaneously. Different sports describe angular movement using terminology that fits sporting contexts and usually has origins in long traditions. Although it is perfectly acceptable to talk about angular motion in terms of degrees, the more common approach used in biomechanics is to refer to angular motion in terms of radians. Angular speed and angular velocity are terms used similar to their linear counterparts. Angular acceleration works in the same way as linear acceleration. Angular acceleration is the rate at which angular velocity changes with respect to time. Or, angular acceleration is the final angular velocity minus the initial angular velocity per unit of time. Since angular velocity, acceleration and other quantities is vector quantities, the right-hand thumb rule can be applied to all of these.

Angular Kinematics of Walking and Running

Many researchers have reported on how the lower extremity joint angles vary throughout the walking and running stride, particularly during the support portion of the stride. An angular kinematic analysis of walking and running typically includes a graphical presentation of joint actions as a function of time. Although some researchers have studied patterns of angular velocity and acceleration in both running and walking, the major focus of investigation has been on the characteristics of angular positions and displacements at critical events in the locomotion cycle. For both walking and running, the greatest range of motion occurs in the sagittal plane, and segment movements in this plane are often used to describe gait characteristics. The calculation of sagittal plane angles can be accomplished with a 2D analysis. However, movement in the other planes can be as critical to successful gait, but obtaining these angles requires a 3D analysis.

Lower Extremity Angles

Although there are obvious magnitude differences where the angular displacements increase with speed of locomotion, the patterns are similar across the speeds of locomotion with some temporal phasing differences. The one exception is at the ankle joint, where there is less and less plantar flexion at heel strike as locomotion speed increases until a point in very fast running at which plantar flexion may be absent.

As contact is made with the ground in both walking and running, a loading response absorbs body weight. The angular kinematics that accompany this response are hip flexion, knee flexion, and ankle dorsiflexion. As the body continues over the foot in midstance, these movements continue until the terminal stages of stance, where there is a reversal into hip extension, knee extension, and plantarflexion.

The initial touchdown hip flexion angle for walking and running has been reported to be in the range of 35° to 40° and 45° to 50°, respectively. In the early phases of contact, the hip adducts in the reported range of 5° to 10° and 8° to 12° for walking and running, respectively. After touchdown, the amount of hip flexion reduces over the course of the support until toe-off, at which 0° to 3° of hip extension in walking and 3° to 5° of hip extension in running is reported. There is also hip movement into abduction at toe-off in the range of 2° to 5° for both walking and running. When the limb is off the ground in the swing phase, hip flexion maximum values are reported in the range of 35° to 50° for walking and 55° to 65° for running. Hip abduction in the initial portion of the swing phase is similar for walking and running, reported to be in the range of 3° to 8°. Hip adduction late in the swing phase varies more between walking and running, in the range of 0° to 5° and 5° to 15°, respectively.

The knee angle is flexed at touchdown and has been reported in the literature to be in the range of 10° to 15° for walking and 21° to 40° for running. After touchdown, the knee flexes to values ranging from 20° to 25° for walking and 38° to 60° for running, with the greater flexion occurring at faster speeds. The knee flexion movement helps to lower the body in stance. Maximal knee flexion occurs at midstance, after which the knee extends until toe-off. Full extension is not achieved at toe-off; values range from 10° to 40° in walking and 18° to 40° in running, depending on speed. Greater extension values at toe-off are generally associated with faster speeds. In the swing phase, knee flexion is important to shorten the swing leg before the hip flexion brings the limb forward. The range of knee flexion in walking and running is reported to be in the range of 50° to 65° and 100° to 125°, respectively.

Again, although the magnitude of the knee angles at these specific instants in time during the support phase of running vary, the profile of the curve does not. The profile of the knee joint angle appears to be relatively stable and immune to distortion from influences such as running shoe construction or delayed-onset muscle soreness.

In walking, the ankle is plantarflexed in a reported range of 5° to 6° at heel strike and moves into 10° to 12° of dorsiflexion before returning to 15° to 20° of plantarflexion at toe-off. During the swing phase of walking, the foot continues on through 18° to 20° of plantarflex-ion and then dorsiflexes in a reported range of 2° to 5° in preparation for the next heel strike. As the speed of locomotion increases, there is less plantarflexion at heel strike until dorsiflexion is the movement occurring at touchdown. Depending on the speed, the reported range of dorsiflexion at heel strike in running is 10° to 17°, increasing to 20° to 30° in midstance and then moving to plantarflexion at toe-off (range, 10° to 20°). Plantarflexion continues into the initial phases of the swing phase (range, 15° to 30°) and then moves, as in walking, into dorsiflexion in the reported range of 10° to 15°.

Alterations in the angular kinematics of the lower extremity joints during both walking and running occur in response to changes in the environment. For example, when running over a noncompliant surface, some individuals make a kinematic adjustment at impact by responding with more initial knee flexion at contact. Walking uphill brings about a number of adjustments in the lower extremity. For example, increasing the grade from 0% to 24%, the lower extremity adjustments start at heel strike with a 22% increase in dorsiflexion, 31% more knee flexion, and 23% more hip flexion. Over the stance phase, there are unequal adjustments at the three lower extremity joints, with the hip joint undergoing the greatest increase in the range of motion (+ 59%), followed by the ankle (+ 20%) and an actual decrease (-12%) range of motion at the knee. The primary adjustment to walking downhill during the stance phase occurs at the knee joint, where there is as much as 15° more knee flexion in early stance. Movement adjustments in the swing phase occur at the hip and ankle, with less hip flexion and less plantarflexion.

Rearfoot Motion

A number of investigations have described the rearfoot angle during the support phase of walking and running. Excessive rearfoot motion during running has been hypothesized to cause a variety of lower extremity injuries, although little evidence directly relates excessive rearfoot motion and injury. In fact, a valid, clinical definition of excessive rearfoot motion has not yet been determined. From a functional standpoint, eversion of the calcaneus is necessary because it allows the foot to assume a flat position on the ground. Typically, maximum rearfoot angle values from -6° to -17° at midstance have been reported in the literature for running and in the range of -9.2 to -12.9° for walking. This wide range in maximum values can be attributable to differences in the anatomical foot structure of individuals as well as the influence of footwear. It has been reported that more extreme rearfoot angles occurs at midstance in running when the subjects wear racing shoes compared with training shoes. More extreme rearfoot eversion angles have also been reported for runners in a shoe with a very soft midsole than in a shoe with a firmer midsole. Although the rearfoot angle is related in motion to the knee angle by the action of tibial rotation, it is, unlike the knee angle, highly variable and certainly can be influenced by many factors.

The simultaneous actions of these two lower extremity angles has been a topic of several investigations. Because internal tibial rotation accompanies knee flexion and subtalar joint eversion and both reach a maximum at mid-stance, the mistiming of these joint actions has been suggested as a possible mechanism for lower extremity injury. Hamill et al. illustrated that the rearfoot angle could be changed by a running shoe with a very soft midsole, but the knee angle could not. These researchers reported that in a soft midsole running shoe, the maximum rearfoot angle occurs sooner in the support period than did maximum knee flexion. The subtalar joint also stays at this maximum while the knee begins to extend. Thus, they surmised that a twisting action may be applied to the tibia by the differential speeds at which the tibia rotated early in support and late in support. Because the tibia is a rigid structure and may be difficult to twist, the tibia may continue to rotate internally at the knee, even though it should externally rotate. This undesirable action at the knee may possibly cause knee pain in the runner. If these actions are repeated with each foot-to-ground contact and the runner has many foot-to-ground contacts, the runner may be subject to a knee injury that would prohibit training. This type of injury is often referred to as an overuse injury. It results from an accumulation of stresses rather than a single high-level, traumatic stress.

Clinical Angular Changes

Locomotion is also influenced by a variety of medical conditions and functional limitations. For example, the walking gait of an individual with Parkinson's disease usually exhibits small, quick steps and less range of motion in the lower extremity joints. A tight hip flexor (e.g., psoas muscle) in individuals with cerebral palsy can limit the hip extension during the stance phase. This causes an increase in pelvic tilt. Specific adjustments in the joint kinematics of individuals with hemiplegia may show a reduction in the range of motion at the knee joint, with increases in range of motion at the ankle and excessive hip and knee motion in the swing phase. Finally, individuals with injury to one limb typically compensate for pain in one limb by altering range of motion in both limbs so they can increase the time spent on the limb with no pain.

Angular Kinematics of the Golf Swing

The linear speed and path of the club head are important determinants of a successful golf shot. These two linear kinematic components of the swing are the result of a series of angular movements; thus, the angular kinematics of the golf swing is commonly the primary focus of golf instruction and evaluation. The golf swing can be accurately described using a double pendulum model, with one link being the arm rotating about the shoulder joint and the second link being the club and wrist, where the wrist acts as a hinge about which the club rotates. A third connected link has been suggested between the shoulder and what is referred to as the hub axis as the body rotates about a vertical axis. For purposes of this introduction to the golf swing, the primary focus will be on the double pendulum characteristics of the swing.

In a golf swing, the left arm (for a right-handed golfer) sets the plane of the swing. The swing plane is an elliptical plane around the body that brings the club head into contact with the ball from the inside, where the face of the club ends up perpendicular to the flight path of the ball. The swing is a pivot about an axis running through the base of the neck with the head stationary. Many beginning golfers try to create an upright swing plane with the club brought straight back and straight forward. When the club head comes down to meet the ball with this swing plane, it is never square with the ball and puts spin on the ball at contact.

The angular positions of the club at various stages of the swing are good predictors of a successful swing. A frontal view of the golf swing provides a good perspective for evaluating club position. In the first stage of the swing, the golfer addresses the ball. This position at the beginning of the swing should be the same as the position at impact. It establishes the arm and shoulder position that will bring the club into precise alignment for impact. The club and the left arm should form a straight line, and the club face should be aimed down a perpendicular line from the ball forward in a straight line. As the club is started in the backswing, there is an initial takeaway phase where the club head is taken back away from the ball. This is initiated with a weight shift to the rear that allows for greater range of motion at the hip and flattens the arc of the swing. A long takeaway is preferred: The club travels in a wide arc, and the wrist does not allow movement of the club until the hands are chest high. This increases the distance for the club head to travel as the shoulders are rotated farther from the target. At the end of the takeaway phase, the left arm should be horizontal to the ground, and the club should be vertical and perpendicular to the arm. Continuing to the top of the backswing, the upper body has rotated to allow the club to be positioned parallel to the ground again and parallel to the final target line for ball contact. The right elbow flexes at the end of the backswing to reduce the length and allow for more acceleration. The left arm continues to be straight and vertical. This position ensures that the club face will travel squarely to the ball at contact. From the top of the backswing, the downswing begins as the club shaft and the left arm drop in one piece to the position halfway down, where the left arm is again parallel to the ground and the club is vertical. Hip rotation and the legs initiate this movement as they drive forward, dropping the right shoulder and the shaft into place. The impact position should duplicate the initial address position, with the left arm and club forming a straight vertical line and the club face traveling in a straight line through the ball. If these angular positions can be obtained within the context of a fluid swing, the ball will travel far and accurately.

The interaction of the arm and club links are shown in the displacement, velocity, and acceleration curves in the downswing phase. The displacement of the arm segment in the downswing is 100° to 270°, and the displacement of the club relative to the arm is 50° to 175°. As the shoulder displacement increases in the early phases, the wrist angle remains constant until it uncocked in the later stages of the downswing. This uncocking increases dramatically 80 to 100 ms before impact as the club is brought in line with the hands. The interaction between the arm and the club segments enhances the velocity and acceleration of the club at impact. This is illustrated in the angular velocity graph, where the arm velocity moves through a range of 250°/s, increasing to 800°/s and reducing velocity to 500°/s at impact. The resulting effect on the club segment is a build in velocity from zero initially to a culminating 2300 to 4000°/s at impact. Angular accelerations of the club are minimal in the beginning of the downswing and increase rapidly to values approaching 10,000°/s/s at a point where the angular acceleration of the arm is reduced to zero and begins the negative acceleration.

Angle and Angular Displacement

Angles express mutual orientation of lines, planes, or a line and a plane. For example the axis of shin and the axis of thigh represent two intersecting lines. The mutual orientation of these two lines can be expressed by an angle. We often need to know the angle between individual body segments to describe, evaluate, and improve skills in physical exercise and sport.

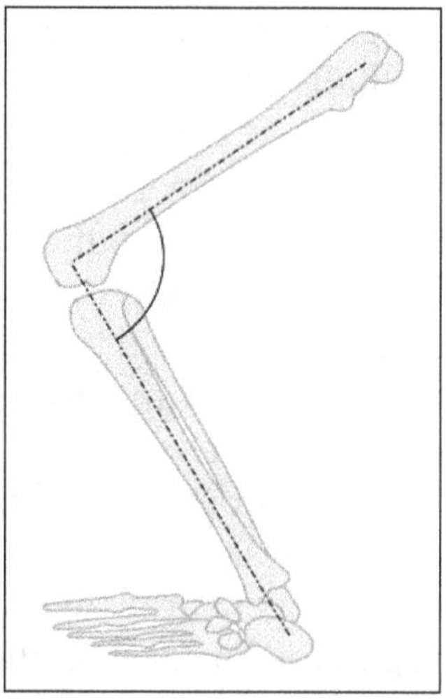

Intersecting axes of shin and thigh during squat and leap upward produce an angle.

Angle and Position

If one of the lines or planes is in a fixed position with respect to the ground, the mutual position of lines or planes is called absolute angle. For example the angle between shin and a fixed horizontal plane is an absolute angle. If both lines, or planes, move relative to each other, we are talking about relative angles. Angles measured in individual joints of human body are angles that describe the relative mutual position of individual parts of human body. Angles (planar angles) are measured in radians (rad). It holds true that a planar angle, which is at the same time a plane, has the size 2π rad. Mathematically an angle can be defined as:

$$\varphi = \frac{l}{r},$$

where φ is planar angle (rad), l is the length of a circular arc, centred at the vertex of the angle (m) and r is the radius of the circle (m).

Angular Displacement

Angular displacement is used to express the extent of motion in individual joints of human body. Angular displacement is the change of the absolute angle between the initial and the final position of a given segment of human body. In biomechanics we usually describe angular displacement between individual segments of human body. We can imagine a single point on each segment, connected by a ray with the intersection of these two segments (i.e. the joint). Change of mutual orientation of these rays equals angular displacement.

Angular displacement is the change of the absolute angle between the initial and the final position of a given segment of human body.

Angular displacement is a vector and its vector line lies in the axis of rotation with counter clockwise direction. We can also use the right-hand rule: if the thumb of our right hand shows the correct direction of angular displacement vector in the axis of rotation, the fingers show positive direction of rotation. Therefore we always try first to identify the plane of motion and the axis of rotation. The axis of rotation is always perpendicular to the plane on which the motion takes place. For example knee flexion takes place in sagittal plane and transversal axis. How then is angular displacement measured? Let us try to measure the extent of knee flexion. At the beginning of the measurement the initial position of shank in relation to the vertical axis is 5°. In the lowest squat position the position of shank in relation to the vertical axis is 45°. Angular displacement $\Delta\varphi$ is then calculated as:

$$\Delta\varphi = \varphi_{\text{final}} - \varphi_{\text{initial}}$$

$$\Delta\varphi = 45 - 5$$

$$\Delta\varphi = 40^\circ,$$

where φ_{final} is the final angle of shank in relation to the vertical axis (rad) and $\varphi_{initial}$ is the initial angle of shank in relation to the vertical axis.

During handspring in gymnastics we have to carry out a wrist motion in large enough extent to give maximum vertical velocity to our body. The number of turns in somersaults that we can see in gymnastics, freestyle skiing, or diving, is a measure of angular displacement and is a very important criterion for the overall result in a given sport. Backward swings in certain gymnastics elements, such as roll into swing, must be described with the angle of backward swing. Iron cross in gymnastics is also assessed with the use of angular displacement. Angular displacement of a swing in football, tennis, golf, etc. has a substantial influence on the resulting stroke into a projectile.

Angular Displacement, Distance and Displacement

When we use ice hockey sticks, tennis rackets, golf clubs, etc., we make longer otherwise short distances our arms would have travelled without using these instruments. Try to imagine elbow flexion when lifting a weight: our hand travels about ten times longer distance than the insertion of our biceps brachii. Distance travelled l of any point of a rotating body is in direct proportion to the angular displacement $\Delta\varphi$ and the radius of the circle r along which the motion takes place:

$$l = \Delta\varphi r.$$

The fact that insertions of our muscles are very near to the axes of our joints brings an important benefit, as it is becoming clear now. Muscles can thus contract over shorter distance to effect longer distances of motion of our extremities. The length of muscle contraction is limited to 50 % of their original rest length. For this reason extremities' motions would be increasingly limited with the growing distance between the axis of rotation and the muscles insertion.

Angular Velocity

Mean angular velocity ω (rad/s) is calculated as the change to angular displacement $\Delta\varphi$ from its initial $\varphi_{initial}$ to final φ_{final} value over time Δt during which the change occurred:

$$\omega = \frac{\Delta\varphi}{\Delta t} = \frac{\varphi_{\text{final}} - \varphi_{\text{initial}}}{\Delta t}$$

Angular velocity is a vector quantity and its direction is specified by the right-hand rule. The SI unit of angular velocity is radian per second (rad/s).

If, however, we are interested to know how fast a body rotates at a certain instant, we describe this by instantaneous angular velocity. With the help of mean angular velocity of a tennis racket stroke we can calculate whether a tennis player is going to hit the ball. Instantaneous angular velocity of a tennis racket at the moment of a stroke (i.e. contact with the ball) determines the following velocity of the ball. In sports such as gymnastics the more important factor of performance is mean angular velocity because it determines how many somersaults and twists the given athlete can manage.

Angular velocity is a ratio of the change of angular displacement and the time during which the change occurred.

Relation between Angular Velocity and Peripheral Velocity

In tennis, golf, hockey, and other sport events the instruments used make our arms longer. If, in these sport events, we tried to toss the projectile using only our arms, we would never achieve such velocity as we do after strokes with a hockey stick, tennis racket, golf club, etc.

The magnitude of peripheral velocity of any point on a rotating body equals the product of angular velocity of that body and the radius of the circle along which that point is moving.

$$v = \omega r,$$

where v (m/s) is the magnitude of peripheral velocity of any point of the body rotating along a circle (e.g. velocity of the hockey stick blade at the moment of contact with the puck), ω (rad/s) is the instantaneous angular velocity, and r (m) is the radius of the circle.

Velocity of a point lying further from the axis of rotation is higher than that of points lying nearer to the axis. Angular velocity of all points of a given body is the same, however. For example longer golf clubs are used for driving with higher initial velocity to longer distances. Shorter golf clubs are used for shorter distances. If we hold a tennis racket at the very end of its handle, we can produce the highest peripheral velocity of its functional end and thus the highest initial velocity of the ball after the stroke.

In sports there is an important concept of effective radius. Effective radius is achieved not only with the length of athlete's arm and the length of an instrument but also with the overall technique of the stroke execution.

The relation between peripheral and angular velocity provides us with a theoretical basis of understanding why the specific arrangement of human muscles and their insertions, in relation to the axis of rotation in given human joints, gives us such an advantage. For example our feet move much faster than is the speed of muscle contraction in those muscles that control the motion of legs in walking and running.

Angular Acceleration

Angular acceleration, also called rotational acceleration, is a quantitative expression of the change in angular velocity that a spinning object undergoes per unit time. It is a vector quantity, consisting of a magnitude component and either of two defined directions or senses.

The magnitude, or length, of the angular acceleration vector is directly proportional to the rate of change of angular velocity, and is measured in radian s per second squared (rad/s ^{2} or rad · s $^{-2}$). Alternatively, the angular acceleration magnitude can be expressed in degrees per second squared (deg/s ^{2} or deg · s $^{-2}$). The direction of the angular acceleration vector is perpendicular to the plane in which the rotation takes place. If the increase in angular velocity appears clockwise with respect to an observer, then the angular acceleration vector points away from the observer. If the increase in angular velocity appears counterclockwise, then the angular acceleration vector points toward the observer.

The angular acceleration vector does not necessarily point in the same direction as the angular velocity vector. Consider a car rolling forward along a highway at increasing speed. The angular acceleration vectors for all four tires point toward the left along the lines containing the wheel axles. If the car stops accelerating and maintains a constant velocity, the angular acceleration vectors disappear. If the car slows down going forward, the vectors reverse their directions, and point toward the right along the lines containing the wheel axles. If the car is put into reverse and increases velocity going backwards, the angular acceleration vectors point toward the right along the lines containing the axles. If the backward velocity is constant, the angular acceleration vectors vanish; if the backward velocity decreases, the angular acceleration vectors point toward the left along the lines containing the wheel axles.

Angular acceleration is the rate of change of angular velocity over time. Mathematically we can define mean angular acceleration as:

$$\omega = \frac{\Delta\varphi}{\Delta t} = \frac{\varphi_{\text{final}} - \varphi_{\text{initial}}}{\Delta t}$$

where ε (rad/s²) is mean angular acceleration (rad/s²), Δω is the change of angular velocity(rad/s), Δt (s) is the time during which the change of angular velocity Δω occurred, ω_{final} (rad/s) is the angular velocity at the end of the studied process, and $\omega_{initial}$ (rad/s) is the angular velocity at the beginning of the studied process. Angular acceleration is measured in radians per second squared (rad/s²).

Angular acceleration is generated when the speed of rotation of a body increases or decreases, or if the axis of rotation changes its orientation.

Angular Acceleration, Tangential Acceleration, Centripetal Acceleration

If the magnitude of angular velocity ω grows, peripheral velocity v also grows. It implies that there is a relation between angular acceleration ε and tangential acceleration a_t.

Tangential Acceleration

Acceleration of any point of a rotating body can be resolved into two perpendicular components: Tangential and centripetal. The tangential component (the tangent to the circular trajectory of a given point) is called tangential acceleration a_t. The magnitudes of tangential acceleration and angular acceleration are interrelated:

$$a_t = \varepsilon r ,$$

where a_t (m/s^2) is the magnitude of tangential acceleration, ε (rad/s^2) is the magnitude of angular acceleration, and r (m) is the radius of the circumscribed circle.

Tangential acceleration is a component of acceleration and it has the direction of the tangent to the circular trajectory.

Centripetal Acceleration

Even if a body rotates with a constant angular velocity, non-zero acceleration results. This acceleration is related to the change in the direction of peripheral velocity of any point of a rotating body and it is called centripetal acceleration a_d. If we imagine what force we have to exert in order to change the direction of a carving turn in downhill skiing, we can realize the direction of centripetal acceleration. Our lean, as well as the forces that incurvate the trajectory of our downhill motion, are directed towards the centre of our ski turns. According to the Newton's second law, centripetal acceleration appertained to these forces is also directed towards the centre of our ski turns. Mathematically the magnitude of centripetal acceleration can be defined as:

$$a_d = \frac{v^2}{r}$$

or also

$$a_d = \omega^2 r$$

where a_d (m/s^2) is the magnitude of centripetal acceleration, v_t (m/s) is the magnitude of tangential velocity of a point of the rotating body, r (m) is the radius of the circumscribed circle, and ω (rad/s) is angular velocity.

Centripetal acceleration is a component of acceleration and it is directed towards the centre of the trajectory's curvature, perpendicularly to the axis of rotation.

The magnitude of centripetal acceleration of any point of a rotating body is directly proportional to the square of angular velocity and the radius of trajectory. If, for example, we are running in the first track, we have to exert greater centripetal force and thus accelerate towards the centre more than if we are running in the last track. For this reason the friction between track shoes and the surface is greater if we are running in the first track. In this case our tangential velocity is the same, only the radius of the trajectory is different. For thinking about centripetal acceleration we used the equation $a_d \frac{v_t^2}{r}$ because our tangential velocity is the same in both cases.

Let us imagine a hockey player with two hockey sticks of various lengths. Both sticks have approximately the same weight but their length is different. What force must the hockey player exert with these two different sticks during a slap shot, if he keeps the same angular velocity? In this case we will calculate centripetal acceleration with the use of the equation $\boldsymbol{a}_d = \omega^2 r$ because the player's tangential velocity is the same in both cases. The player must exert greater force and greater centripetal acceleration when using the longer stick (r in this case is the perpendicular distance of the stick's centre of gravity from the axis of rotation). We must realize, however, that even though the longer stick is better for shooting with higher initial velocity, the player must exert greater force to achieve that velocity compared to using the shorter stick. If the stick is too long, the player might not even be able to achieve sufficient velocity of the shot.

Movement Patterns

Basic movement patterns are realistically just a way of categorising exercises based on their biomechanical demands. Classifying exercises into these categories makes it easier for the strength and conditioning coach to identify which exercise is most appropriate for the athlete.

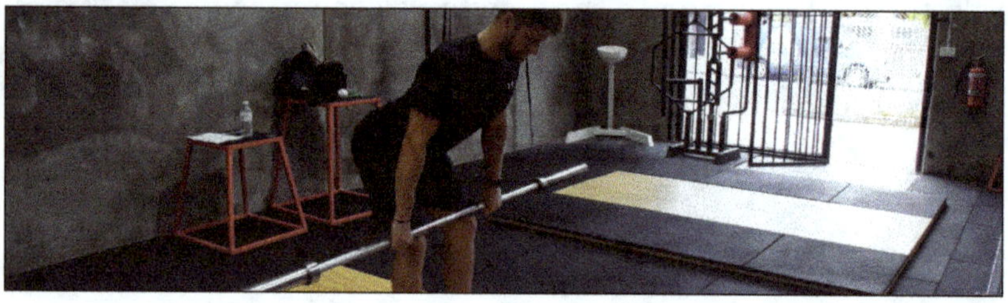

For decades gym-based training has revolved around the concept of training muscle groups in isolation. Though nobody knows exactly, it is commonly agreed that this very concept has stemmed primarily from bodybuilding. However, strength training pioneers such as Prof. Yuri Verkhoshansky and Dr. Michael Yessis began to popularise gym-based training for athletes during the mid-20th century. Since then, global developments on how to train athletes, and how to make it functional for their sport has accelerated – particularly in recent years. Perhaps these advancements are associated with the immense commercial growth of sport and thus the increase in sports science related degrees and courses worldwide. Regardless, strength and conditioning coaches and exercise specialists all over the world now appreciate the significant difference between training athletes and training others (e.g. bodybuilders).

Basic Movement Patterns

Basic exercise movement patterns are, quite simply, exercise classifications, which due to popularity have formed the foundations of exercise selection. Once a strength and conditioning coach determines which basic movement patterns are essential for the athlete, they will they devise a battery of exercises forged from those movement patterns (i.e. exercise classifications). For example, a primary movement pattern of a rowing athlete is a horizontal pulling action, as a result, a 'horizontal pulling' movement (e.g. Prone Rows) may become a vital component of their training programme. On the other hand, a leg extension exercise would be classified as a 'knee dominant' movement, as the knee joint is the prime lever. Although there are thousands of different exercises, a large majority of them can be categorised into the following movement patterns.

- Hip Hinge.
- Hip Dominant.
- Knee Dominant.
- Vertical Push.
- Vertical Pull.
- Horizontal Push.
- Horizontal Pull.
- Rotational and Diagonal.
- Anti-rotation.
- Anti-flexion.
- Anti-extension.
- Anti-lateral Flexion.

Classification

At present, this is normally done by anecdotal evidence and purely based on the opinion of the strength and conditioning coach and their scientific knowledge of each exercise. However, there are common rules of thumb that are followed to categorise each exercise. These are segregated by one of three things:

- The movement direction of the exercise (e.g. flat bench press is a horizontal press).
- The primary joint lever (e.g. during the knee extension, the knee joint is the primary lever).
- Or, by the joint deemed to experience the largest 'relative' forces (e.g. let's just suggest that the hip is capable of handling higher joint forces than the knee. During a pistol squat, whilst the forces exerted on the hip may be larger than those on the knee, the knee might be enduring its maximal tolerance. In which case, this may be deemed as a knee-dominant movement because the knee is experiencing the largest 'relative' forces). Note that this is purely a fictitious example.

Examples of the basic movement patterns:

Hip Hinge

This category of exercises is comprised of exercises that involve a hinging motion at the hip joint, with little to no knee movement. These hip dominant exercises are initiated by a contraction of the hip extensors (e.g. glutes, hamstrings) and spinal erectors to extend the hip. These exercises tend to be more of a pulling action as opposed to a push.

The following are examples of hip hinge exercises:

- Romanian Deadlift (RDL) and its variations (e.g. single-leg).
- Kettlebell Swing.

Hip Dominant

Though this category can include hip hinging movements, it is used to identify all exercises in which the hip joint plays the primary role. For example, whilst the Glute Bridge is a hip dominant movement, it is not reflective of a hip hinging movement. Similarly, the High-Box Step-up is also a hip dominant movement that is not reflective of a hip hinge.

The following are examples of hip dominant exercises:

- Glute Bridges.
- High-box Step-ups.
- Leg Press (position-specific).
- Romanian Deadlift (RDL) and its variations (e.g. single-leg).
- Kettlebell Swing.
- Squat (Bilateral variations) However, this is really a misnomer as it is not really either knee or hip dominant -it's both.

Knee Dominant

This category is classified by movements in which the knee is the dominant lever during the exercise.

The following are examples of knee dominant exercises:

- Single-leg Squats (Pistol, Bulgarian, Knee-tap, Elevated).
- Low-box Step up.
- Lunge (Forward, Backward, Lateral).
- Leg Press (position-specific).

- Squat (Bilateral variations) However, this is really a misnomer as it is not really either knee or hip dominant -it's both.

Vertical Push

This category of exercises include all exercises that move the load/weight vertically in relation to the torso, or at least in that direction. It usually consists of movements in the sagittal plane (shoulder flexion) or frontal planes (shoulder abduction). Furthermore, this normally means its movements create shoulder abduction and flexion and extension of the elbow (i.e. pushing).

The following are examples of vertical push exercises:

- Push Press.
- Military Press.
- Overhead Dumbbell Press.
- Seated Shoulder Press.
- Jammer Press.

Vertical Pull

This category of exercises also includes moving a load/weight vertically in relation to the torso, or at least in that direction. However, it usually consists of movements in the sagittal (shoulder extension), frontal, or transverse planes (shoulder adduction). Furthermore, this normally means its movements create shoulder extension and adduction with elbow flexion (i.e. pulling).

The following are examples of vertical pull exercises:

- Pull-ups (Close-grip, Wide-grip, Supinated-grip etc).
- Lat Pull-downs.
- Kneeling Pull-downs.
- Plank Rows.

Horizontal Push

This category of exercises involves moving a weight straight out in front of you, away from the torso. Therefore, it consists of movements in the sagittal (shoulder flexion) and transverse plane (shoulder horizontal adduction) with elbow extension (i.e. pushing).

The following are examples of horizontal push exercises:

- Press-ups.

- Bench Press.
- Standing Chest Press.
- Single-arm Dumbbell Press.
- Kneeling Single-arm Press.

Horizontal Pull

This category of exercises involves moving a weight towards the torso. Therefore, it consists of movements in the sagittal (shoulder extension) and transverse plane (shoulder horizontal abduction) with elbow flexion (i.e. pulling).

The following are examples of horizontal pull exercises:

- Inverted Row.
- Bench Row.
- Bent Over Row (Bilateral, Unilateral, Barbell, Dumbbell, Kettlebell etc).
- T-bar Row.
- Seated Row.
- Kneeling Single-arm Row.

Rotational and Diagonal

This category of exercises are primarily associated with movements of a rotational nature, typically within the transverse plane. These movements may also incorporate some form of pushing and pulling movements.

The following are examples of Rotational/Diagonal exercises:

- Russian Twist.
- Barbell Torque.
- Cable Rotations.
- Woodchops.
- Lateral Medicine Ball Throw.

Anti-rotation

Anti-rotation exercises are designed to challenge the lumbo-pelvic complex muscles (i.e. the core) to prevent rotation in the transverse plane and improve stiffness and stability of the spine – hence the term 'anti-rotation'. Some exercises in this category also fall into other categorises, meaning some exercises can have dual purposes and therefore potentially more 'bang for your bucks'.

The following are anti-rotation exercises:

- Horizontal Palov Press.
- Single-arm Dumbbell Chest Press.
- Single-arm Rows.

Anti-flexion

Anti-flexion exercises are designed to challenge the lumbo-pelvic complex and spinal erector muscles to prevent flexion and improve stiffness and stability of the spine–hence the term 'anti-flexion'. Most exercises in this category are associated with common exercises and therefore they are not often referred to as anti-flexion.

The following are anti-flexion exercises:

- Squat.
- Deadlift.
- Bent Over Row.

Anti-extension

Anti-extension exercises are designed to challenge the lumbo-pelvic complex and spinal flexor muscles to prevent extension in the sagittal plane and improve stiffness and stability of the spine– hence the term 'anti-extension.

The following are anti-extension exercises:

- The Plank and its variations.
- Press-ups.
- Supermans.
- Crocodile Crawls.
- Commando Crawls.

Anti-lateral Flexion

Anti-lateral flexion exercises are designed to challenge the lumbo-pelvic complex and spinal erector muscles to prevent lateral flexion and improve stiffness and stability of the spine – hence the term 'anti-lateral flexion.

The following are anti-lateral flexion exercises:

- Vertical Palov Press.
- Single-arm Overhead Press.
- Imbalance Lunges.
- Imbalance Step-ups.
- Imbalance Farmer Walks.

Kinetic Link Principle

The kinetic link principle (KLP) refers to the method in which the body produces momentous force. A summation of forces is produced through the body via a 'linking' process of a number of segments together. Diagram produced by Kreighbaum describes a sequential process by which a force is produced. It describes force starting from the proximal segments of the body and progressively transferring momentum to the distal segments. This is possible via the proximal segments being larger in mass and having a greater inertia. An upper body throwing action may be used as an example. The initial segments (i.e. trunk rotators) accelerate eliciting a force, where the next body segment (i.e. shoulder horizontal adductors/internal rotators) then initiates an accelerating force, which then refers on to the upper arm (i.e. elbow extensors), and the end point (wrist and finger flexors). The key to this process is that each segment is smaller than the previous and contains less inertia. As one segment accelerates it allows the following segment to initiate movement at its top speed as it passes on momentum to the next segment before it decelerates. The speed of the consecutive segments gradually increases, with the result allowing the end point velocity of the final segment to be much greater than the initial. This biomechanical process occurs through the "serape/functional line effect" and can be applicable to not only a throwing action, but a range of different functional skills.

Subijana performed a biomechanical study on kinetic energy transfer during the tennis serve. They analysed two tennis player's service actions via a system referred to as 3D photogrammetry, where a proximal to distal segment kinetic energy transfer was discovered by a mean correlation analysis. The analysis found that for one of the players it could successfully predict the quality of the serve with 100% accuracy and the other player 76%, based on the kinetic transfer properties seen during the action.

Roetert referred to a tennis serving action. He reported the following findings:

- The largest portions of kinetic energy or force generated in the serving stroke are developed in the legs and trunk, where 51% of the kinetic energy and 54-60% of the total force are produced.
- As seen in diagrams, each segment has a cocking or stabilization phase, and an acceleration phase.

- Segment 'drop out' or kinetic chain breakage decreases the ultimate force and energy available to produce a forceful movement, and also puts excessive unnecessary strain on the surrounding segments.
- A 10% reduction in energy transferal from the hip or trunk requires a 14% increase in shoulder rotation velocity or a 22% increase in shoulder mass to create the same amount of kinetic energy for the movement.

The KLP is a very trainable aspect of functional development where analysis of the process one uses to efficiently accelerate at different joints can be identified, and exercise prescription can be applied to enhance the method of force transferal through the body. This process is common in a number of sports such as baseball, golf and tennis, where biomechanical feedback is given to the individual athlete so alterations can be made to decrease the potential for injury occurrence and improve the power profile through one or more specific sporting actions.

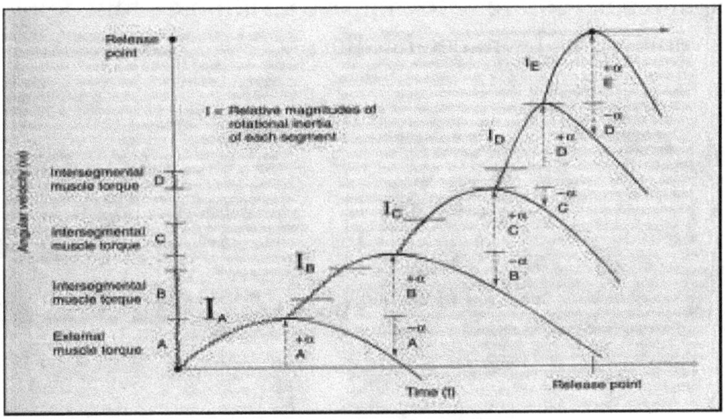

Kinetic link principle.

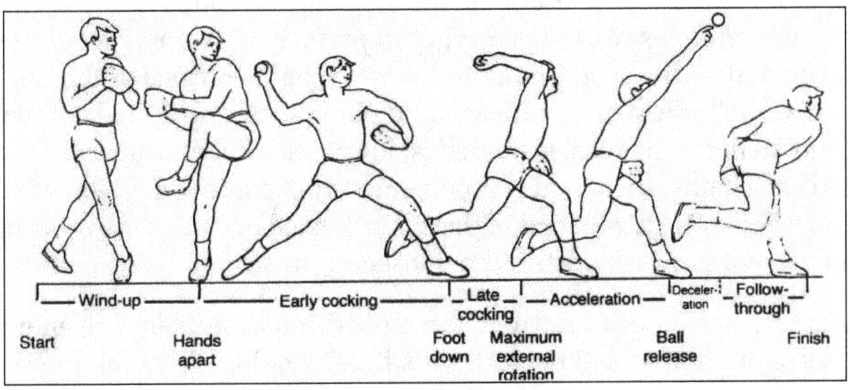

Kinetic link principle in action.

The order of recruitment of muscles combined with using the correct amount of elasticity at the right time determines how much momentum and "end point" force is generated. An effective throwing arm in softball, a spike in volleyball, or a kicking action in football all come down to the specific order of actions an athlete uses to produce force.

A simple explanation can be used in a sporting example. In javelin a throwing action begins with the legs. The athlete uses the lower body initially to extend the legs (the largest muscles), then the trunk to extend and rotate (moderate size muscles), then the throwing arm for release (smaller muscles), in a specific order to generate momentum to produce maximal force and power into the action.

Overall strength in the individual muscles is a factor but far from a determining one. The primary issue is that the order of recruitment and coordinated effect of the movements are in the correct sequence. If there is a problem throughout any part of this sequence such as an inactive/weak muscle (such as the gluteals) or hypertonic (tight) muscles or soft tissues (fascia/tendon) it creates an ineffective link in the chain, where load and momentum is not dispersed evenly and effectively, so ease of movement and power generation is not as great.

The KLP is very trainable for all athletes of all sports, where a functional strength training coach and a skills coach combine to improve an athlete's functional deficits to allow improvement movement for their specific sport.

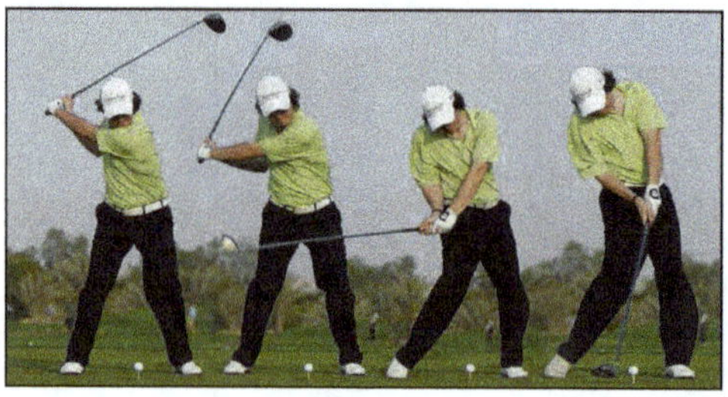

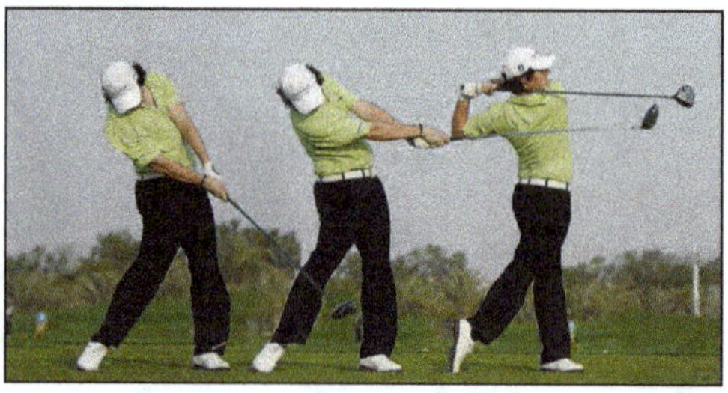

Kinetic Chain

Anatomically, the kinetic chain describes the interrelated groups of body segments, connecting joints, and muscles working together to perform movements and the portion of the spine to which they connect. The upper kinetic chain consists of the fingers, wrists, forearms, elbows, upper arms, shoulders, shoulder blades, and spinal column. The lower kinetic chain includes the toes, feet, ankles, lower legs, knees, upper legs, hips, pelvis, and spine. In both chains, each joint is independently capable of a variety of movements. Dependent on whether the distal end of the chain is fixed or free to move without restriction, each movement is classified as either closed or open.

A closed chain refers to a position where the most distal aspects of a given extremity are fixed to the earth or another solid object. This fixed position alters the movement of the joints and surrounding musculature up the chain. For example, if the feet are planted on the ground during a squat, the rest of the leg chain (i.e., ankles, knees, and hips) will move toward the fixed end of the extremity—the feet—as the body lowers into the squatting position. In contrast, an open chain refers to the distal end of an extremity moving freely in space—such as when performing a biceps curl with dumbbells or a seated leg extension on a weight machine—where the movement of the distal end of the extremity is not fixed.

Closed-chain movements promote joint stabilization and have the potential to recruit more muscles and their associated joints. Further, closed-chain movements are transferable to many daily movements that involve more than one joint, which may lead to better neuromuscular coordination and overall joint health. Thus, many closed-chain exercises are considered "functional" and used in programming for functional training purposes [i.e., purposeful exercise that trains movement—not isolated muscle groups—and intentionally incorporates balance and body awareness (proprioception)].

Open-chain movements, in contrast, involve more shearing forces at the involved joint compared to closed-chain movements and tend to recruit the musculature associated with only a single working joint in resistance training exercises like leg extensions and biceps curls.

Examples of closed-chain exercises include:

- Squat,
- Wall slide,
- Lunge,
- Push up,
- Pull up.

Notice that in each of the above exercises the distal end of the extremity is fixed, which results in the body moving about the fixed joint.

Examples of open-chain exercises include:

- Seated leg extension,
- Leg curl,
- Bench press,
- Dumbbell biceps curl,
- Lat pull-down.

Notice that in each of the above exercises the distal end of the extremity is not fixed, and it moves about the body during the movement.

Fluid Mechanics

Fluid mechanics or fluid dynamics comes into sport a lot and covers air resistance, drag, projectiles, spin on balls and Bernoulli principle and lift force.

Spin

Spin is created by applying a force that is off centre to the object being thrown (or kicked) at the point of release. The effects of spin are important in all ball sports and throwing events. The Magnus effect explains why the paths of balls deviate from normal flight path.

Projectiles

A projectile is anybody who is thrown or jumped into the air. Once it has left the ground it will follow a flight path called a parabola until it once more comes back down to earth. This applies to balls, javelins, discus, long jumpers, high jumpers, and horses show-jumping.

Bernoulli Principle

The Bernoulli principle explains why aeroplanes fly and racing cars stick to the ground going around corners when they really shouldn't. It is to do with lift force and down-force created when air flows over an aerofoil.

Air Resistance and Drag

Air resistance is a frictional force that occurs when air passes over the surface of a body. This frictional force is not just limited to air though and it applies in fluids, usually water in a sporting situation. Air resistance, drag, and fluid resistance mean the same thing.

Buoyancy

An object's ability to float in a liquid depends on the density of the object compared with the density of the fluid in which the object is immersed. Water exerts pressure equally in all directions, even upward. You can feel the upward force (buoyancy) of water when you try to push something under the water. Buoyancy results from the difference in pressures on the upper and lower surfaces of an object. The weight of an object plus the weight of the fluid (air, water, or both) above the object exert a downward force. Fluid pressure pushes upward from below. The difference between these two forces is the buoyancy of the object.

Archimedes, an ancient Greek scientist, discovered that the force of buoyancy acting on a submerged object equals the weight of the water displaced (this is known as Archimedes' principle). A hot-air balloon floats in air because the hot air inside the balloon weighs less than the volume of cooler air the balloon occupies. A diver is buoyed upward with a force equal to the weight of the water that the diver displaces. If you and your equipment weigh less than the weight of the water you displace, you will float, or have positive buoyancy. If you and your equipment weigh more than the water being displaced, you will sink. An object that sinks has negative buoyancy. If you and your equipment weigh exactly the same as the water displaced, you neither float nor sink. Instead, you remain at the depth where you are; you have neutral buoyancy.

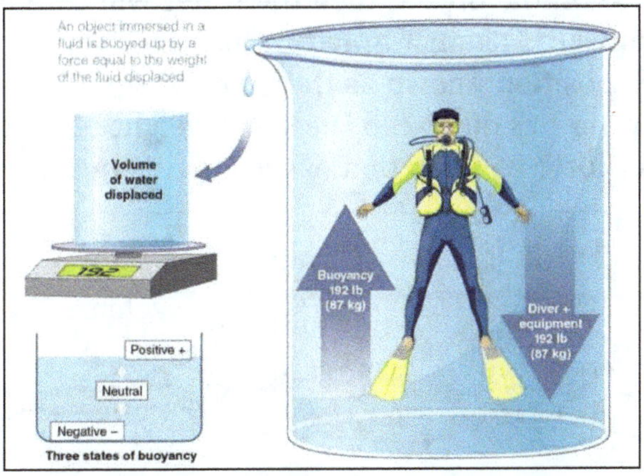

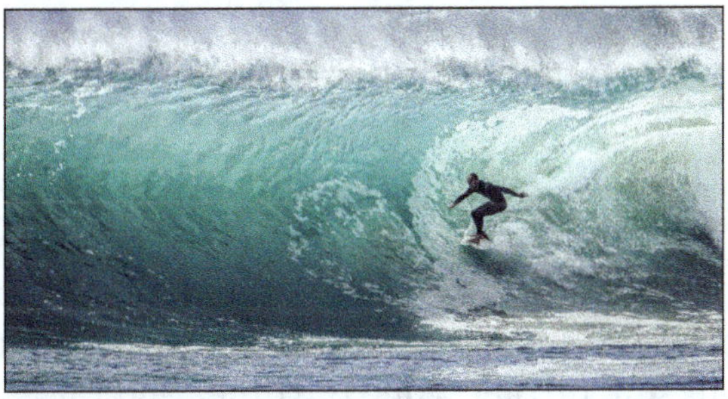

The first dash point under fluid mechanics is flotation, centre of buoyancy. These two concepts are put together because floatation is caused by a force known as buoyancy. For an object to float in water it must be less dense (mass per unit of volume) than the water.

When an object is placed in water it causes the water to be displaced (move upwards). This can be seen when a person gets into a bath and the water rises. If the bath is filled to the very brim, then when the person gets into the bath the water that is displaced will pour out of the tub. In order for an object to float, the water they displace must weight more than they do.

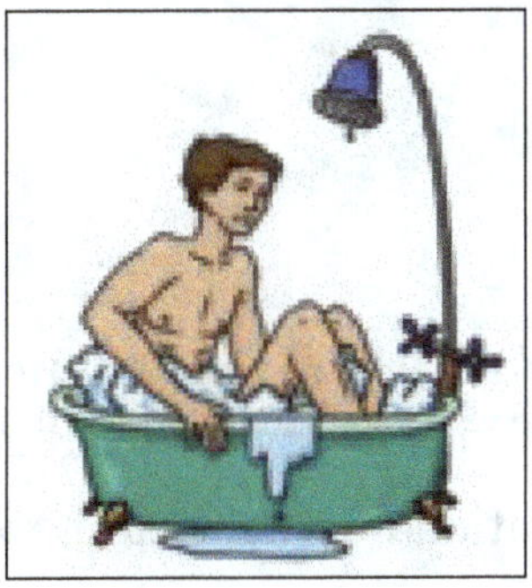

In order for an object to float, the water they displace must weight more than they do. This is essentially because gravity is seeking to push the water that has been displaced, back down, while also pushing the person down. If the gravitational force on the water is greater than the force on the object, then the water will create a buoyant force that will push the object upwards against gravity. Once the two forces become equal the object will float in this position known as the point of equilibrium. That is the part of the object below the water has displaced the same weight of water, as the object itself, resulting in a bouyancy force equal to that of the gravity force acting on the object.

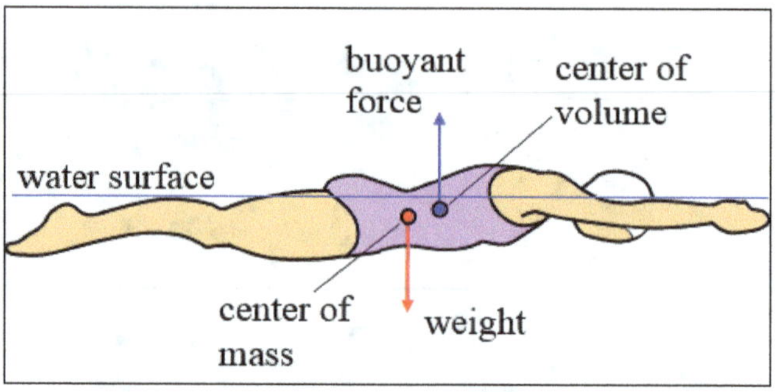

The centre of buoyancy is the centre point of the mass below the water and is the point through which the buoyant force acts. This is much like the centre of gravity – the point through which gravity acts, but buoyant forces acts in the opposite direction. In order for the object to not rotate in the water this buoyant force must pass through the center of mass of the object, if they do not line up the object will rotate until they do, such that one end of the object will sink further while the other end raises.

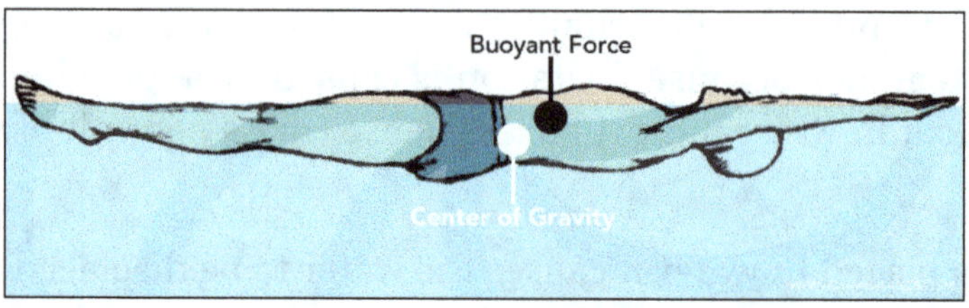

The centre of buoyancy and the centre of gravity do not line up, meaning their will be rotation.

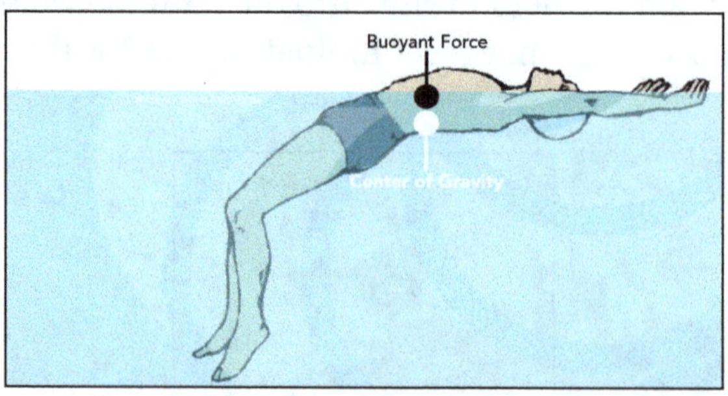

Here they do line up, due to the lowering of the legs into the water and the rising of the chest.

For an object to have less gravitational force than the water it displaces it must be less dense (mass per unit of volume) than the water. Not all water has the same density though. Salt water is more dense than fresh water, and the saltier it is the larger the density. This means that it is easier to flow in the ocean than it is in a pool.

Flotation and centre of buoyancy relate to performance because the higher an object floats in the water, the less resistance the water will create to its movement. This applies to all water sports, including: surfing, kayaking, sailing, skiing, dragon boat racing, water polo, synchronised swimming, and swimming. These forces also relate to scuba diving, where the person is seeking to sink below the water and remain submerged. In this instance, the person, with their gear, wants to be the same density as the water in order to allow them to remain submerged easily, but not have to fight too hard to return to the surface. This is often achieved using weight belts.

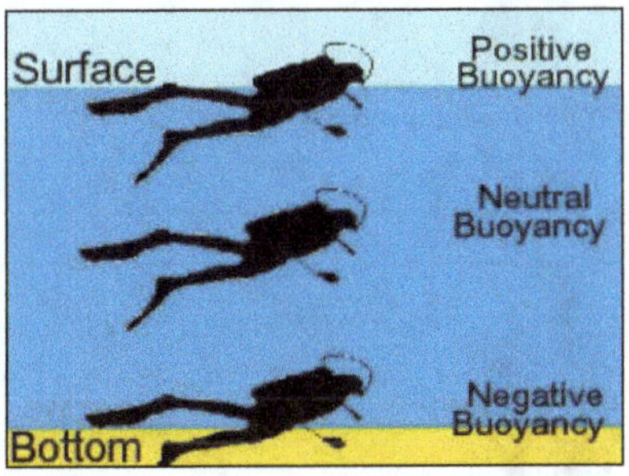

Some examples of modifications that have occurred to take advantage of buoyancy include the Speedo LZR Racer suit, which trapped air making the swimmer more buoyant, lifting them higher in the water so that they had less drag from the water and increased their speed, reducing their times in events.

Other modifications include the change in surfboard technology, where they used to be made out of wood, surfboards are now made of polyurethane or polystyrene covered in fiberglass, and polyester. This creates a lighter surfboard that is more buoyant and maneuverable in the water.

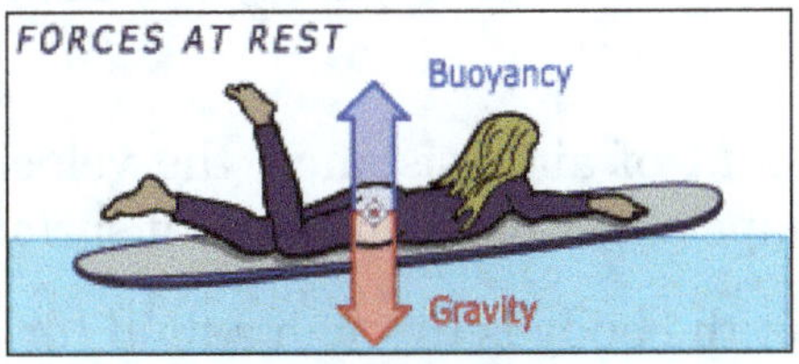

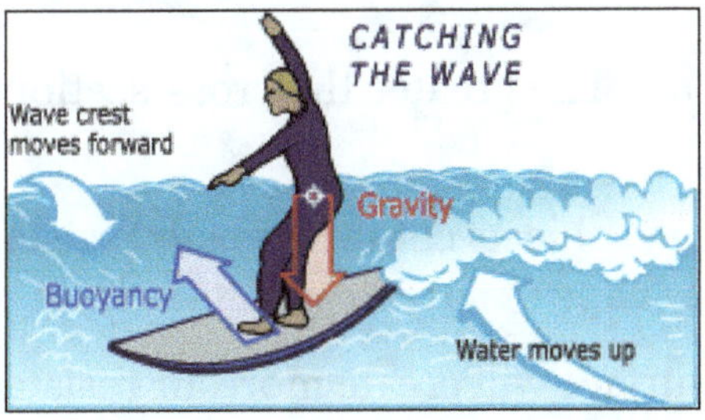

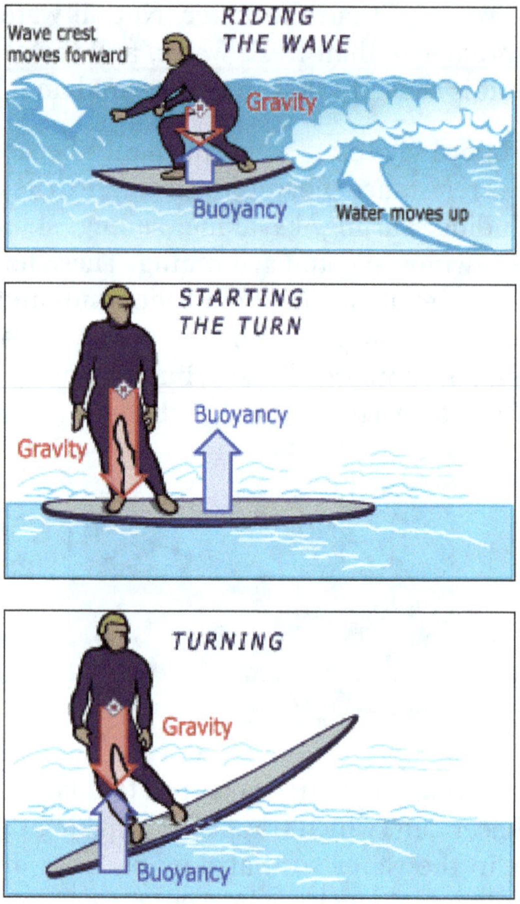

Air Resistance and Drag

Air resistance is a frictional force that occurs when air passes over the surface of a body. This frictional force is not just limited to air though and it applies in fluids, usually water in a sporting situation. Air resistance, drag, and fluid resistance mean the same thing.

Four things affect the amount of air resistance; the velocity of the body or air, the cross-sectional area, the shape of the body and type of surface.

- Velocity – The faster the body is through a fluid (or air), the greater the air resistance.
- Cross-sectional area – The greater the cross-sectional area the greater the air resistance.
- Shape – Pointy shaped objects cut through air resistance more easily, for example, an F1 car or the shape of a track cyclists helmet.
- Surface – A rough surface will create more air resistance or drag than a smooth

surface. Remember the Speedo LZR full-body swimsuit which significantly enhanced a swimmer's performance by holding the body in a more aerodynamic position and repelling water from the surface? The dimples on a golf ball actually decrease air resistance making a golf ball fly further through the air than a smooth ball.

Aerofoil

An aerofoil is a streamlined shape which minimises cross-sectional area and drag of air passing around it.

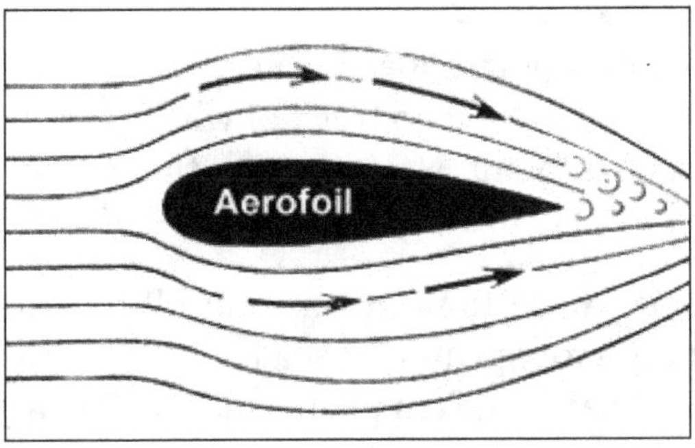

Each sport has its own challenges. Things like air resistance and clothing can separate one athlete from another, or even force the athlete to adapt to a new situation, rejecting the familiar feel of a honed technique, built up in muscle memory.

Speed skating is a good example. The altitude at which a speed skating event is held plays a large factor in the time that it takes to complete the race. In a venue in Sochi, which is near sea level, the air resistance is much greater than it is at a few thousand feet above sea level. This is why all current world records, men's and women's, were set at tracks in Calgary, Alberta, and Salt Lake City, Utah.

But reducing air resistance is a many-headed monster. Air resistance also influences the skaters' posture.

Crouch

Robert the deeply bent, compact tuck position speed skaters use while racing is very uncomfortable. They use that position in order to reduce their air resistance. But, they have to find a way to be able to skate and move their legs at the same time.

"Think about being in a squat, with your leg muscles contracted like they do for 10, 15, 18 minutes. It's an incredibly uncomfortable position to be in, but they've trained for it and it ends up where they can end up doing what they do at amazing levels.

The crouch that speed skaters maintain during a race is so extreme that they reduce blood flow to their legs. "It's only when the leg is extended and the muscles relax, that basically blood is allowed to flow in. It's incredible to look at how much that blood flow gets cut off, but that's the position they have to be in to minimize drag".

In fact, training on the ice is so intense that speed skaters do much of their training somewhere else.

Speed skaters, even though they could be on ice all year around, they don't because it's just so demanding to be in the skating position and go around a curve at 50 kilometers per hour [about 31 mph] that they just can't do that all the time.

Speed Differences

Like so many Winter Olympic sports, speed skating is highly technical. While the athletes are in the crouch, they need to keep track of where they are on the course. Speeding through the turns can be difficult. Now imagine that the same full-out effort results in a different speed based on the altitude of the competition venue.

Male speed skaters average more than 30 mph in all but the longest races, and top women often average 30 mph for sprints. At sea level they might travel 0.5 mph less, or even slower, than they would at a track in places such as Calgary and Salt Lake City, due primarily to the increased air resistance. That means the skater might be going more than 2 percent slower at lower elevations. This could create some difficulty for athletes who train at a higher elevation than at Sochi.

They're going to take those turns at different speeds. One is the speed that they practice at if they've been at altitude and the other is the speed they're going to have when they're at sea level. "Now their speed is going to be a little slower, so their timing is going to end up being just a little bit different." From a motor control or neuromuscular standpoint, they have probably spent time practicing at the competition altitude to avoid errors.

However, many of them probably trained at high altitude, as do many endurance athletes, including cross country skiers, in order to encourage their bodies to produce more red blood cells.

That's helpful for endurance exercise because now you can deliver more oxygen to the muscles, both at altitude and at sea level. "It's a very, very large effect on performance".

Air Resistance beyond the Oval

Effects due to air resistance can even extend to sports where speed is not the main objective. Chapman mentioned figure skating and ski jumping in particular. A figure skater encounters air resistance when trying to make a triple or quadruple jump. Chapman said that rotational speed of a figure skater might be slower at sea level, not much more than a couple of degrees, but he said that being off by that much can make a difference.

The ski jump at the 2014 Winter Olympics is not in Sochi itself, but about 40 miles away, at the mountain venue near Krasnaya Polyana, so jumpers aren't facing the same air resistance as they would at sea level. Air resistance determines the optimum angle for a ski jumper as he or she leans over the skis in order to best form a wing-shape during their flight. The difference between jumping at sea level and at 7,000 feet is more than four degrees of lean.

Sport Aerodynamics

In sports events, performance analysis is not an easy task since multiple factors, such as physiology, psychology, biomechanics, and technical progress in equipment are simultaneously involved and determine the final and ultimate outcome. Identification of individual effects are thus complicated, however from a general point of view, aerodynamics properties are recognized to play a determinant role in almost every sports in which the performance is the result of the optimal motion of the athlete (multi-jointed mechanical system) and is equipment (solid system) in the air. From ball games like golf, baseball, soccer, football and tennis to athletics, alpine skiing, cross-country skiing, ski jumping, cycling, motor sport and many others, the application of some basic principles of aerodynamic can make the difference between winners and losers.

If the general shape of the athlete/equipment system in terms of postural strategies and equipment customization is not optimized, it can either be made to deviate from its initial path, resulting in wrong trajectories and loss of speed and leading to failure in terms of performance. Coaches should thus be able to assess the aerodynamic efficiency of the motor task performed by the athlete with accuracy and in almost real time. Indeed, quick answers and relevant information can help the athlete to focus on specific aspects of his technical behaviour to improve his performance. So far for this purpose, two solutions are available i.e. dedicated wind tunnel testing or implementation of aerodynamic force models during the athlete training sessions. According to the complexity of sport performance and the necessity of almost real time answers for stakeholders, issue concerning the relevance of aerodynamic force modelling versus controlled experiments in wind tunnel must be discussed. In particular when searching to optimize athletes' performances, what are the advantages to develop and implement aerodynamic models comparing to controlled experiments in wind tunnel and for which purpose?

After a short description of the aerodynamic principles commonly applied in sport to help optimize performance, both approaches (wind tunnel testing and aerodynamic force modelling) to assess the aerodynamics properties of a particular mechanical system: the athlete with or without his equipment. It will among others present a review of particular wind tunnel setting and modelling methods dedicated to specific sports such as cycling and skiing as well as shows in section, how appropriate applications of them can lead to an increase of athletes' performances.

Aerodynamic Principles Applied to Help Optimize Performance in Sport

Athletic performance is a part of a complex frame and depends on multiple factors. For sports such those involving running, cycling, speed skating, skiing where the result depends on the time required to propel the athlete's body and his equipment on a given distance, the performance is largely conditioned by the athlete technical skills. Success then is the outcome of a simple principle i.e. the winner is the athlete best able to reduce resistances that must be overcome and best able to sustain an efficient power output to overcome those resistances.

In most of the aforementioned sports, those resistances are mainly the outcome of the combination of the contact force and the aerodynamic force acting on the athlete. The goal in order to optimise the performance consists to reduce both of them as much as possible.

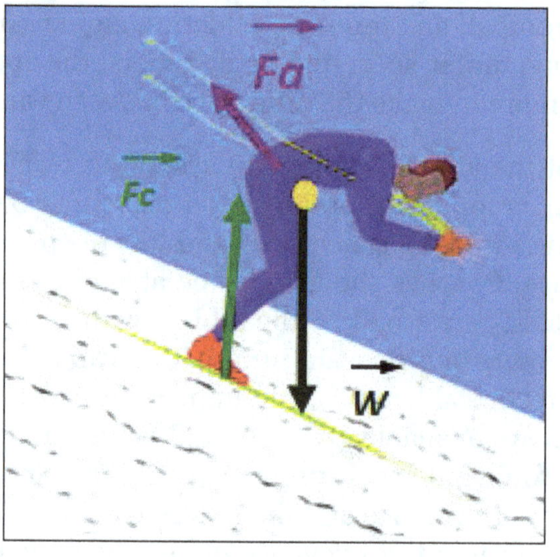

Force acting on a downhill skier. With W ◦ the weight of the skier, Fc◦the ski-snow contact force and Fa◦the aerodynamic force.

However, whether cycling, speed skating, skiing, given optimal physical capabilities, it has been shown that the main parameters that can decreased the race time considerably is the aerodynamic behaviour of the athlete and his equipment. Indeed, in cycling, the aerodynamic resistance is shown to be the primary force impeding the forward motion of the cyclist on a flat track;. At an average speed close to 14 ms^{-1}, the aerodynamic resistance represents nearly 90% of the total power developed by the cyclist. The statement is the same in downhill skiing. The aerodynamic resistance is the parameter that has the greatest negative effect on the speed of the skier. For a skier initially running with a speed of 25 ms^{-1}, the transition from a crouch posture to a deployed posture can induce in 2 seconds (1.8% of the total run) almost a decrease of 12% of the skier speed whereas in the same condition, the ski-snow contact force only lead to a decrease of 2.2%.

It is thus obvious that in such sports where a maximal speed of the system athletes/equipment is needed in order to reduce as much as possible the racing time, an optimisation of the system aerodynamic properties is crucial compare to the optimization of its contact properties.

Fundamentals of Aerodynamic

Aerodynamics in sport is basically the pressure interaction between a mechanic system (athlete and his equipment) and the surrounding air. The system in fact moves in still or unsteady air.

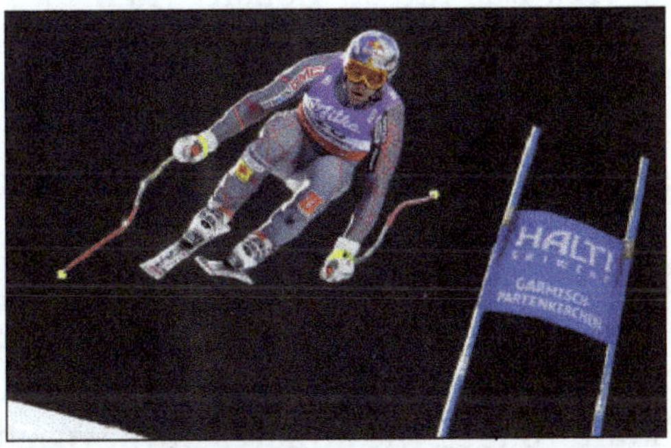

A downhill skier passing over a bump.

By integrating the steady and static pressure field over the system, the resulting aerodynamic force acting on this system can be obtained. This force is generally divided into two components, i.e. the drag force $\overset{o}{D}$ and the lift force $\overset{o}{L}$.

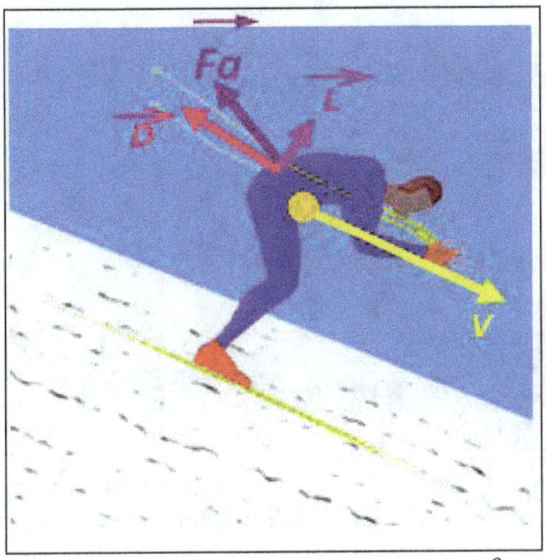

Aerodynamic force applied on a skier and its two components: $\overset{o}{D}$ the drag (axial component) and $\overset{o}{L}$ the lift (normal component). V represents the speed of the skier.

The drag $\overset{o}{D}$ is defined as the projection of the aerodynamic force along the direction of the relative wind. This means that if the relative wind is aligned with the athlete/ equipment system, the drag

coincide with the aerodynamic force opposite to the system motion. $\overset{o}{D}$ depends on three main parameters: (i) the couple athlete/equipment frontal surface area (defined as the surface area of the couple athlete/equipment projected into the plane perpendicular to the direction of motion), (ii) the drag coefficient depending on the shape and the surface quality of the system and (iii) the athlete speed. The drag is thus expressed using the following equation.

$$D = \frac{1}{2} \circ \rho \circ A \circ C_D \circ V^2$$

Where D denotes the drag (N), ρ is the air density (kgm^{-3}), A is the projected frontal area of the couple athlete/equipment (m^2), C_D is the drag coefficient and V is the air flow velocity (ms^{-1}) equivalent to the athlete speed.

The drag is essentially proportional to the square of the velocity and its importance grows more and more as the speed increases. If speed is doubled, the drag increases by four-fold. The drag coefficient C_D is dimensionless and depends on the Reynolds number (ratio ofinertial forcesand forcesduetotheviscosity ofair)andthespeedoftheairflow. If C_D varies for law speed values, in most of the sports considered in this chapter, it can be considered as constant. In fact, the athletes never reach the critical speed which cause the fall in C_D due to the change from laminar to turbulent regime. So at a steady and relatively high speed, variations of drag are mainly induced by variations of the projected frontal area of the couple athlete/equipment, thus by posture variations. The figure shows in which proportion the A.C_D factor of a downhill skier varies with changes in posture.

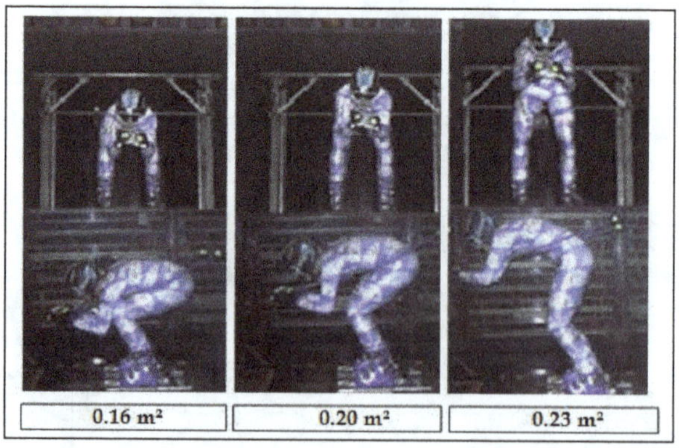

Variation of the A.CD factor of a downhill skier according to posture variations (Wind tunnel of IAT, France).

The lift $\overset{o}{L}$ is the component of the aerodynamic force that overcomes gravity. It is acting normal to the drag component. As the drag, it depends also on three main parameters: (i) the couple athlete/equipment frontal surface area (defined as the surface area of the couple athlete/equipment projected into the plane perpendicular to the direction of motion), (ii) the lift coefficient depending on the shape and the surface quality of the system and (iii) the athlete speed. The lift is thus expressed using the following equation.

$$L = \frac{1}{2} \circ \rho \circ A \circ C_L \circ V^2$$

Where L denotes the lift (N), ρ is the air density (kgm^{-3}), A is the projected frontal area of the couple athlete/equipment (m^2), C_L is the lift coefficient and V is the air flow velocity (ms^{-1}) equivalent to the athlete speed.

Bernoulli's lawexplainsthephenomenonofliftfrompressure differencesbetweenthelower and upper surfacesof theprofileof a mechanical system.

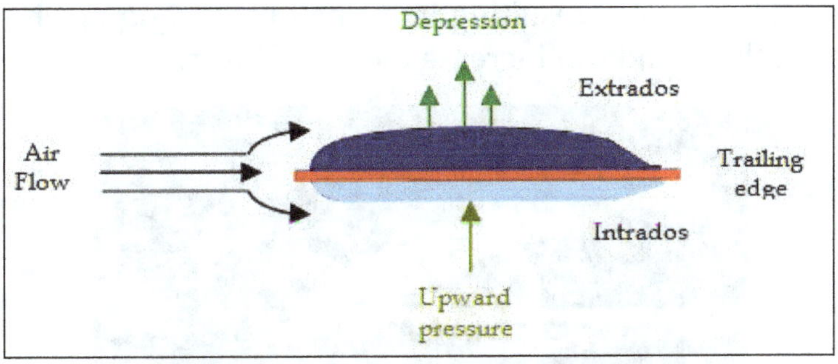

The lift effect according to Bernoulli's law.

The distance travelled by the air flow is more important above the extrados than below the intrados. To avoid creating a vacuum of air at the trailing edge, the air flow following the extrados must move faster than the one following the intrados. An upward pressure is thus formed on the intrados and a depression appears on the extrados, thereby creating a phenomenon of lift. The shape of the mechanical system and its surface quality have thus, an effect on the lift intensity. However in the same manner as the drag coefficient C_D, the lift coefficient can be considered constant for the ranges of speed practiced during the aforementioned sports. Variations of the surface opposing the airflow induced by variations of the angle between the system chord line and the longitudinal axis namely the angle of incidence (i), impact the variability of the lift. For an angle of incidence greater than 0 °, the lift will tend to increase while for an angle of incidence lower than 0 °, a phenomenon of "negative lift" will appear (downforce).

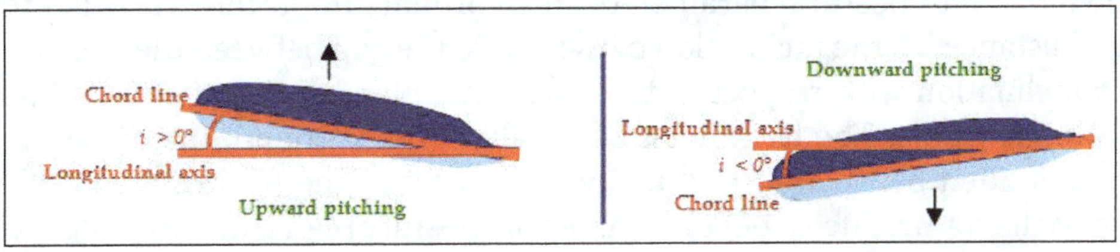

Profile of an object according to its angle of incidence. i correspond to the angle of incidence.

In the aforementioned sports (running, cycling, skiing, skating), the equipment surface is rather small with respect to the athlete surface and therefore the main part of the aerodynamic force acts on the athlete who can be regarded as bluff body (non streamed line body). The bluffness leads to the fact that the aerodynamic resistance is mainly pressure drag instead of friction drag and thus, on a general point of view, it's more important to reduce the frontal area than to reduce the wet area. Then as lift is generally not required, it's better to keep it as small as possible in order to avoid the production of induced drag. However, in particular sport like ski jumping, it is obvious that the flight length is sensitive both to lift and drag. Small changes in the lift and or drag can have important effect for the jump quality and the skier must find the right compromise between an angle of incidence that will lead to an increase of the lift but not to an increase of the drag. The athlete must thus produce an angular momentum forwards in order to obtain an advantageous angle of incidence as soon as possible after leaving the ramp. If the forward angular momentum is too low, the flight posture will induce a high drag thus a law speed and a low lift, resulting in a small jump. Too much forward angular momentum on the other hand can increase the tumbling risk.

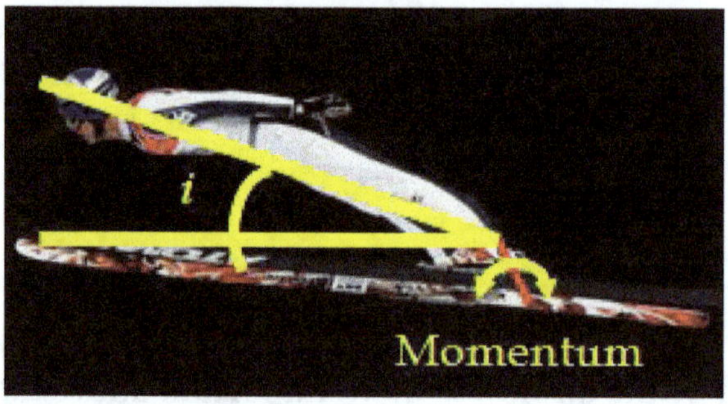

A ski jumper during the flight phase just after leaving the ramp.

Reducing the Aerodynamic Force to Optimize the Performance

Reducing the air resistance in sport events typically involved improving the geometry of the athlete/equipment system. Optimisation of the athlete postures as well as the features of his equipment is generally required since they have a pronounced impact on the intensity of the aerodynamic force.

Firstly, by proper movement of the body segments (upper limbs, trunk, lower limbs) in order to minimize the frontal surface area exposed to the air flow, the posture can become more efficient aerodynamically. For example, in time trial cycling, it is now well known that four postural parameters are of primary importance in order to reduce the drag resistance i.e. the inclination of the trunk, the gap between the two elbows, the forearms inclination with respect to the horizontal plan, the gap between both knees and the bicycle frame. The back must be parallel to the ground, the elbow closed up, the forearms tilted between 5° and 20° with respect to the horizontal and the knees closed up to the frame. Such a posture (time trial posture) can lead to average reduction of the drag resistance of 14,95% compared to a classical “road posture” (37.8±0.5 N vs. 44.5±0.7 N; $p<0.05$)and that merely because of significantly lower frontal area (0.342±0.007 m2 vs. 0.398±0.006 m2; $p<0.05$).

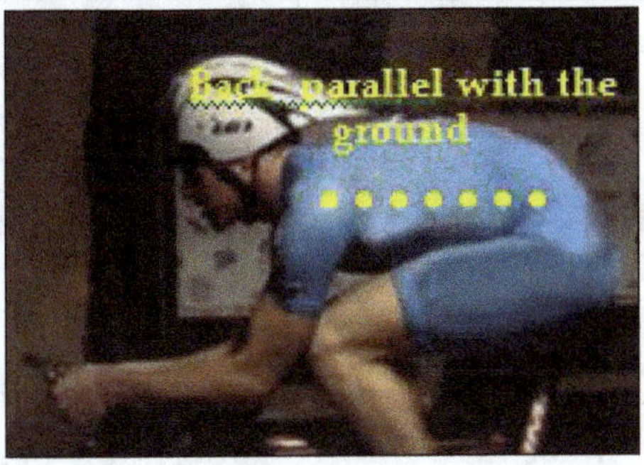

An optimal aerodynamic posture in time trial cycling.

In downhill skiing, the principle is the same. The intensity of the aerodynamic resistance is even lower that the skier adopts a compact crouched posture for which the back is round and horizontal, the shoulders are convex and the upper limbs do not cross the outer contour of the skier and especially do not obstruct the bridge created by the legs.

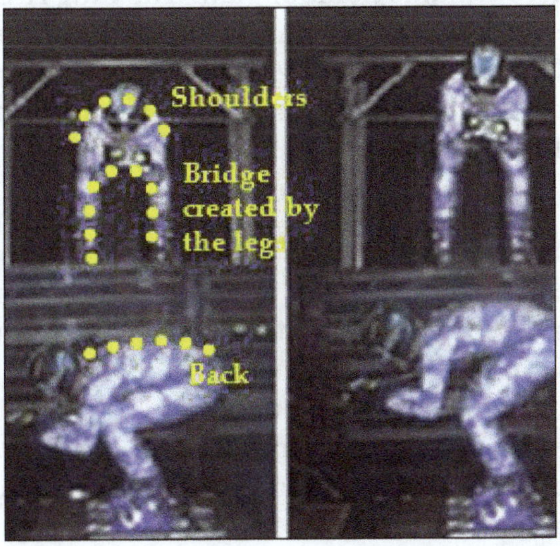

An optimal aerodynamic posture in downhill skiing on the left compare to a posture a little bit more open on the right.

For an initial skier speed of 25ms^{-1}, such a crouched posture can lead to a gain of 0,04 second after a straight run of 100 meters thus to a victory compared to a posture a little bit more open.

Secondly suitable aerodynamic customisation of the equipment can also strongly reduce the negative effect of the aerodynamic resistance. Indeed as example, in cycling, the comparison between time trial helmet and normal road helmet shows a drag resistance improvement that can range from 2,4 % to 4 % according to the inclination of the head.

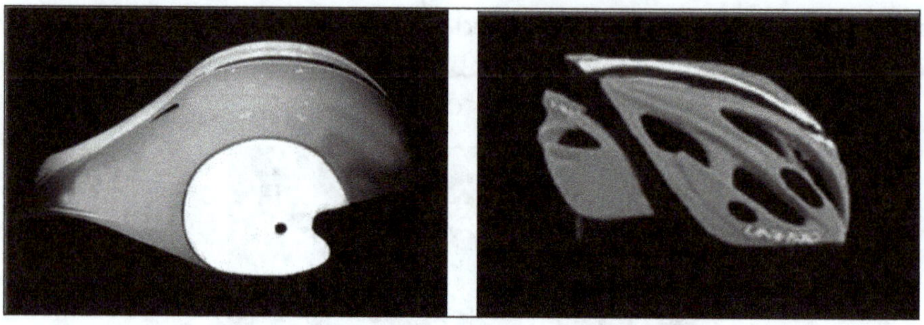

Two cycling helmets, one aerodynamically optimised for time trial event (left) and the other a simple road helmet (right).

It is worth noting that an efficient optimisation of the aerodynamic properties of the athlete/equipment system must take into consideration precisely the interaction between the posture features and the equipment features. The aerodynamic quality of the equipment is totally dependent of the geometry characteristics of the athlete during the sport activity. An efficient optimization cannot be done without taking this point into consideration. In particular in time trial cycling, the interaction between the global posture of the cyclist and the helmet inclination given by the inclination of the head is significant from an aerodynamic point of view. The drag resistance connected with usual inclination of the head is lower (37.2±0.6 N) than the one related to the low slope of the head (37.8±0.5 N), which is itself significantly lower than the one generated by a high slope of the head (38.5±0.6 N). In fact according to the helmet shape, the inclination of the head can have different impact on the projected frontal area of the couple helmet/athlete head thus on the aerodynamic drag.

Hence, it is also important for coaches and athletes to optimize postures in a way that it will not affect the athlete physical power to counteract the resistance. In most of the sport and for aerodynamic purposes, athletes are asked to adopt a tightly crouched posture to reduce their frontal areas exposed to the air stream but if it is not well done, it can also have bad biomechanical and physiological consequences for the athlete performance such as a decrease of physiological qualities. Everything is a compromise. In ice skating for example, although a tightly crouched posture reduces leg power, it reduces air drag to an even greater extent and thus produces higher skating velocities.

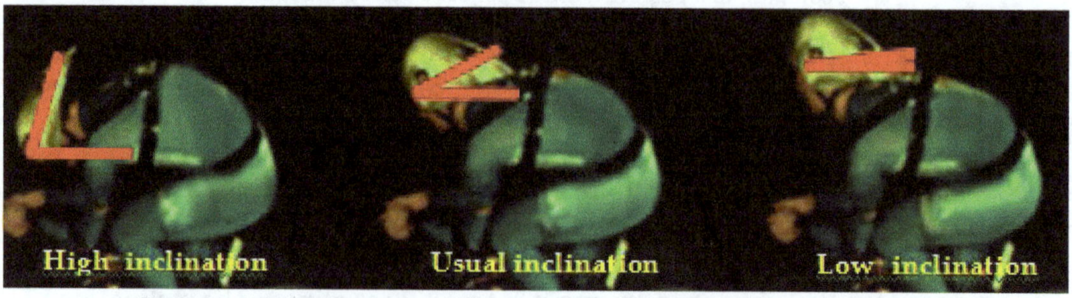

Inclination of the head in time trial and corresponding inclination of the helmet.

Methods for Assessing the Aerodynamic Force Applied on an Athlete with or without his Equipment

To assess the aerodynamic performance of an athlete and his equipment, two methods are available, i.e. either to perform wind tunnel testing to single out only one specific determinant of the performance in this case aerodynamic properties of the athlete or/ and his equipment, or to develop and implement aerodynamic force models that can for example be apply in a real training or competitive conditions which mystifies the role of other factors such as for instance mental factors. The real question here, concern the relevance of the inferences drawn from the results obtain with this two methods according to the fact that the performance in sport is the outcome of the efficient interaction of multiple factors at the right time. Indeed, "a fact observed in particular circumstances can only be the result of particular circumstances. Confirming the general character of such a particular observation, it is taking a risk of committing a misjudgement. Both approaches are further detailed below as well as their relevance according to the performance goal pursue by the principles stakeholders i.e. athletes and coaches.

Wind Tunnel Testing

Wind tunnel tests consist in a huge apparatus used to determine the complex interactions between a velocity-controlled stream of air and the forces exerted on the athlete and his equipment.The tunnel must be over sized compare to the athlete to be assessed in order to avoid side effects that may disturb the measurement of the aerodynamic force. The athlete with or without his equipment is fasten on a measured platform (6 components balance) in the middle of the test section. The athlete is thus stationary in the flow field and the air stream velocity around him generally corresponds to the ones observed during the sport practice (e.g. 14ms^{-1} in time trial cycling, 25 ms^{-1} and more in alpine skiing.). The aerodynamic balance enables to measure the smallest aerodynamic force imposed on the athlete/equipment system in particular its axial (drag) and normal (lift) components.

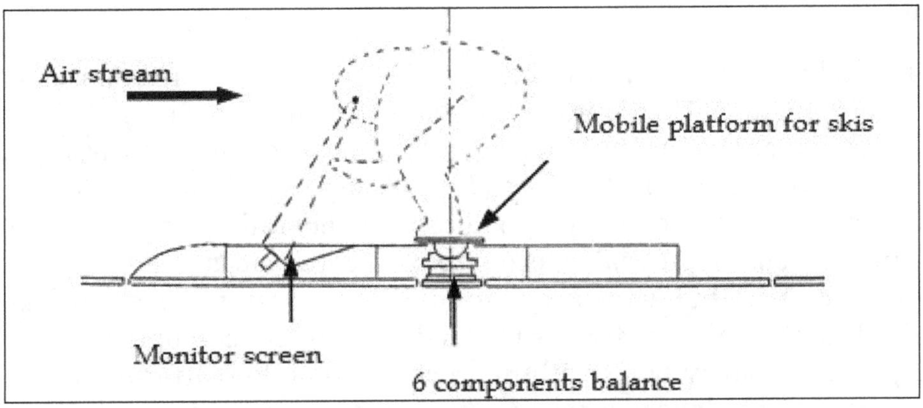

Diagram of a data acquisition system for the assessment of the aerodynamic properties of a downhill skier.

For a better understanding, the path of the air stream around the system can be made visible by generating smoke streams.

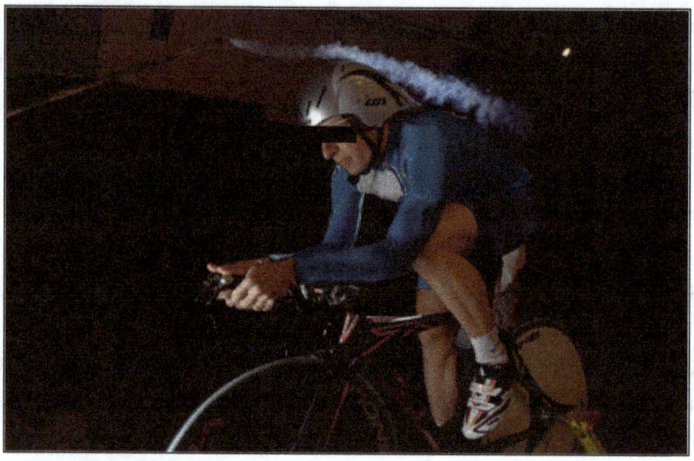

Smoke stream around a time trial cyclist and his equipment.

A tomography gate can also be installed in the wind tunnel behind the athlete to explore the air flow wake behind him.

The figures below shows different wind tunnel settings that have been used for the measurement of the aerodynamic force applied on downhill skiers and time trial cyclists.

In alpine skiing, most of the time, the skier is in contact with the snow and only an accurate assessment of the drag applied on him is necessary. However in particular conditions and especially when he passes over a bump, it is interesting to quantify the lift applied on him. It has to be the smallest as possible since the skier as to be as soon as possible in contact with the snow to manage his trajectory. The length of the jump must be very short according to the initial and following conditions and the goal for the skier is to adopt in the air a posture that will generated the smallest lift. For both purposes i.e. measuring accurately the drag and the lift, two wind tunnel setting must be considered.

On Fig the goal is only to measure the aerodynamic drag applied on a skier adopting a crouched posture. The skier is fastening in the middle of a wind tunnel on a 6 components balance that enables ones to have access to multiple variables, among other the aerodynamic drag. Wind-less balance signals acquisition (during which the skier has to keep the crouched posture) are generally performed before each aerodynamic measurement trial, in order to correct the measurements for zero drift and mass tares. After the zeros acquisition, the wind tunnel is started and when the required speed of the air flow is reached, the athlete can optimized is posture according to the strategy build with his coach. A mobile platform allowed him to adjust the posture of his legs whenever he wants according to the information he can read on the monitor screen.

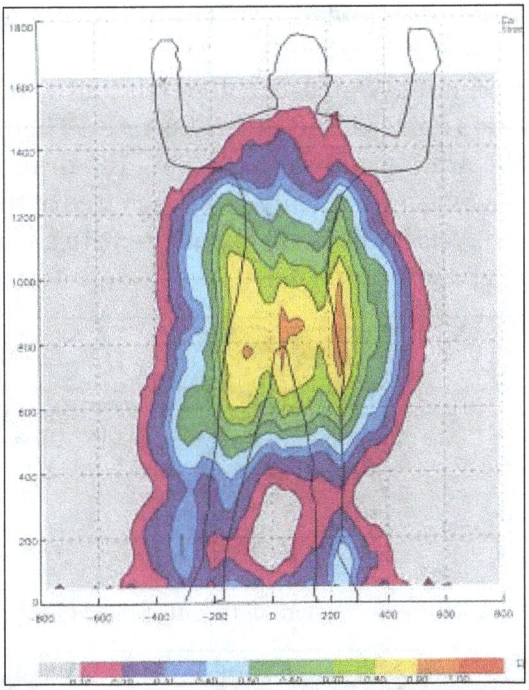

Mapping of the air flow behind a cross country skier. The more colours are warm, the more the aerodynamic resistance is important.

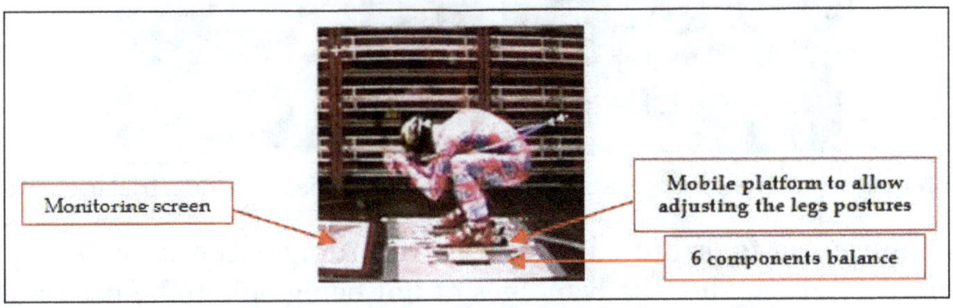

Measuring device for the assessment of the drag applied on a downhill skier.

If the skis have not a great impact on the variability of the drag intensity, their contribution to the variability of the lift has to be taken into account. It is therefore necessary to position the skis outside the boundary layer which is near the ground. Although it is relatively thin, the velocity of the airflow in this area varies significantly and disturbs the measurement of the lift. Sections of boat masts located under each skis have thus allowed to overcome this problem and allowed to remove the skis from this thin layer where the air stream can transit from a laminar to turbulent conditions.

In time trial cycling, in order to determine the drag force of the system bicycle /cyclist, a cycletrainer is fastened on a drag-measurement platform mounted in the middle of the test-section of a wind tunnel which dimensions (octagonal section with inside circle of 3 meters in diameter and 6 meters length) allowed to avoid walls boundary layer effects that can interfering measurements. This platform is equipped with ball-bearing slides in the direction of the wind tunnel as well as a dynamometer measuring the drag force. As for assessing the aerodynamic properties of a skier, the general procedure for a cyclist is the same. A preliminary measurement without wind is performed in order to correct the measurements for zero drift and mass tares. Then a second measurement with wind but without the athlete allowed obtaining the drag force of solely the platform equipped with the cycletrainer. Finally, the drag force of the couple bicycle/cyclist can be measured while the cyclist adjusted his posture with a wind speed similar to that found in race conditions (around 14 ms^{-1}).

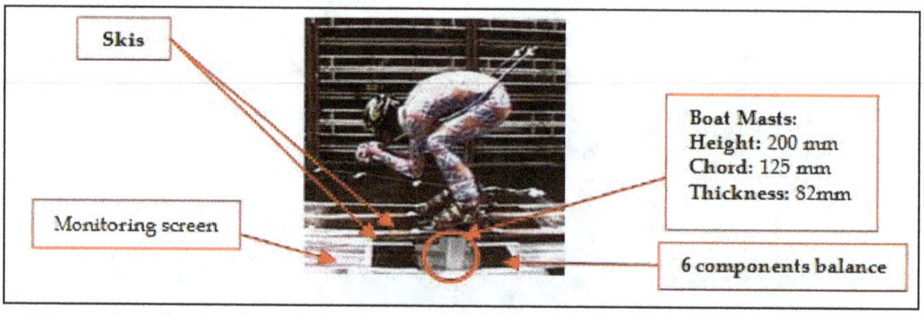

Measuring device for the assessment of the lift applied on a downhill skier.

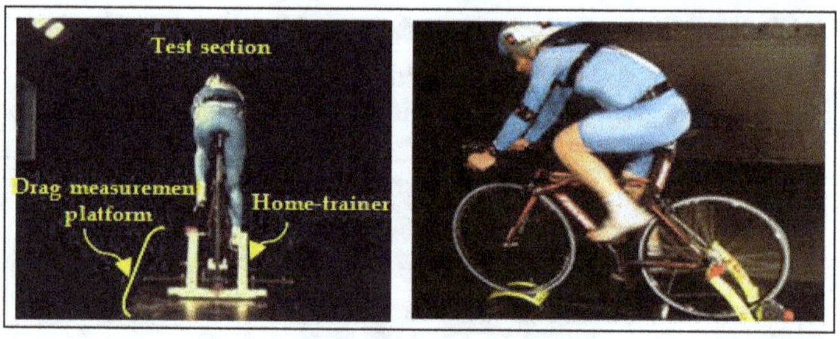

Measuring device for the assessment of the drag applied on a time trial cyclist.

If such a measurement tools provides accurate recording of the aerodynamic force apply on the athlete, it has the disadvantages of not being able to be used anytime it is needed. Specific and dedicated wind tunnel program has to be perform and sometimes far away from the athletes current concerns. Moreover, the usual environmental conditions of the sport practice are requirements that cannot be taken into account in a wind tunnel setting.

Modelling Methods

For numerical models, the method consists in computing correlation between postural parameters observe during the practice as well as equipment characteristics when or if needed and the value of the aerodynamic force. It requires most of the time and previously wind tunnel data of the aerodynamic characteristics of the athlete according to various postures and if necessary within a wide range of orientations relative to the air flow. Indeed, the functions are generally determined with athletes or model of athletes positioned in a wind tunnel in accordance with postures observed during competition in the field.

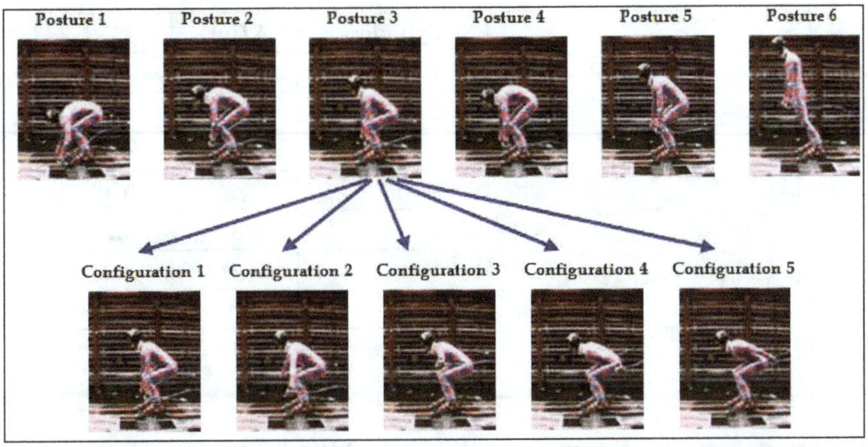

postures assed in wind tunnel prior the development of a model of the aerodynamic lift applied on a downhill skier when passing over a bump. These postures correspond to postures observed in real conditions.

The results of such models can then serve for example as input for simulations based on the Newton laws to estimate variations in time, loss in speed performance induced by different postural strategies as well as equipment interactions. When dedicated simulators integrating such models already exist, an almost real time feedback can be provided to the stakeholder on the aerodynamic properties of the athletes' posture. This can be a cost effective solution since it needs few human and material resources and it can be performed anytime it is needed during normal training sessions.

Examples of the development approach of some models for the evaluation of the aerodynamic performance in running, skiing, cycling are presented and discussed below.

Modelling of the Aerodynamic Force in Running

Have developed a model for the determination of the drag force on a runner. They have considered the human body as a multi-jointed mechanical system composed of various segment and showed that the drag assessment applied on an athlete could be realized by considering the athlete's body as a set of cylinders. Their model is thus composed of a series of conjugated circular cylinders, to simulate the trunk and the lower and upper limbs, as well as a sphere to simulate the head. Projected surface area was measured for each segments (head, neck, trunk, arm, forearm, tight, shank) of the body of three runners representing respectively, adult American males in the 2.5, 50 and 97.5 percentiles of the population. Then the drag coefficient of cylinders and sphere representing these segments has been measured in a wind tunnel. The results for the 50 percentiles are proposed in the table here after.

If such a model has the merit to enable one to reach the drag coefficient of the body segments of a runner, it doesn't consider the athlete body has a whole as well as the succession of body segments orientations that can generate different projected surface area and thus variation of the air resistance throughout the global motion of the runner.

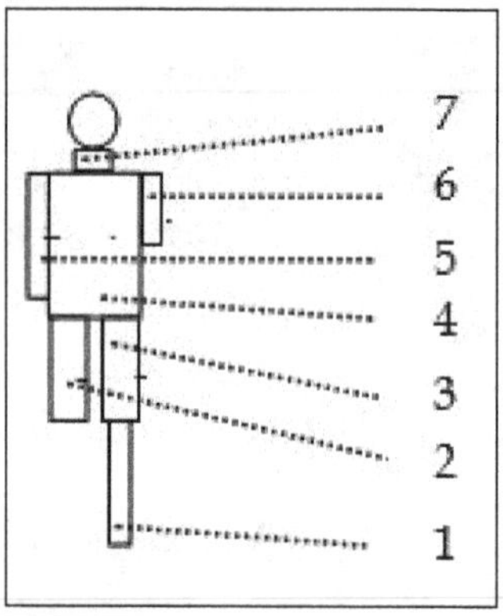

Cylinders	A (in²)	C_D
1	64.5	1.2
2	67.7	1.2
3	67.7	1.2
4	312	1.1
5	78.1	1.2
6	43.2	1.2
7	11	1.2
Sphere	48.3	0.43

Table: Models to determine the drag coefficient of the body part of a runner according to their projected surface area.

Moreover the adaptation of such model to different runners or to different kind of sportsmen during their practice is time consuming and not in accordance with the stakeholders (coaches, athletes) requirement of a quick assessment of the aerodynamic performance of an athlete.

Modelling of the Aerodynamic Force in Skiing

The aerodynamic resistance in alpine skiing has been largely investigated, leading to different approaches to model the aerodynamic force. Have used experimental data obtained in a wind tunnel in their approach of the aerodynamic resistance applied on a skier. They have attempted to assess the influence of aerodynamic and anthropometric speed skier. By combining the three variables most influencing the speed of the skier i.e. his weight, is projected surface area (reflecting its morphological characteristics), and the drag coefficient C_D, they established a numerical code (ACN: Anthropometric Digital Code) representing the aerodynamic characteristics of skiers. The model is written as follow:

$$ACN = \left(\frac{mg}{A.C_D} \right)^{1/2}$$

Where m is the skier mass, A is the projected frontal area, C_D is the drag coefficient.

If the factors mg and C_D (invariable for skiers dressed with the same race clothes) are easily accessible, this model set the problem of assessing the projected frontal area of the skier in real condition. The observer (coaches) because of its placement on the side of the track can hardly have a front view of the athlete in action and even if he had it, it would not allow him to determine directly and easily the A. The model of for the drag and lift lead to the same problem. For this purpose, have developed a an images processing software to determine A but the processing time is once again too important for field application.

Uses the conservation of energy principle in order to model the term $A.C_D$.

$$A.C_D = \frac{m\left(V_D^2 - V_F^2\right) - 2k.V.mg.d}{V^2.d}$$

Where m is the skier mass, A is the projected frontal area, C_D is the drag coefficient, V_D is the initial speed of the skier, V_F is the final speed of the skier, V is the mean speed of the skier, k the snow friction coefficient and the air density, d the distance travelled by the skier.

While this model takes into account as input data, field variables (speed of the skier, travelled distance), it does not incorporate the influence of postures variations. Once again the results obtained from this model can only be an approximation for use in real conditions since it cannot explain with accuracy the performance variations induced by changes in posture.

The modelling of the aerodynamic force as it is described above is not relevant and efficient for rapid application in real conditions. If in straight running, skiers can easily maintained an optimal crouched posture, in technical sections (turns, bumps, jumps), they must manage their gestures to ensure an optimal control of their trajectory, while minimizing the aerodynamic effects. To be relevant for such real conditions applications, posture variations must be taken into account in the modelling and thus whatever the considered sport.

Modelling of the Aerodynamic Force in Cycling

As cyclists' performances depend mainly on their ability to get into the most suited posture in order to expose the smallest area to the air flow action, the knowledge of their projected frontal area can be useful in order to estimate their aerodynamic qualities. By the way, several authors have either reported values of A or developed specific equations to estimate the projected frontal area. However, this has been generally done only for riders of similar size and adopting the same posture on a standard bicycle. Such estimations have then shown large divergences and methodological differences may have widely contributed to such variability. Thus to be useful, models mustn't be developed as black boxes but by indicating accurately why they have been develop for and in which condition they can be used, by being transparent on the variables that have served to its construction and the results accuracy it can provided.

For example, have developed a model estimating accurately A as a function of anthropometric properties, postural variations of the cyclist and the helmet characteristics. From experiments carried out in a wind tunnel test-section, drag force measurements, 3D motion analysis and frontal view of the cyclists were performed. Computerized planimetry measurements of Awere then matched with factors related to the cyclist posture and the helmet inclination and length. A Principal Component Analysis has been performed using the set of data obtained during the experiment. It has shown that A can be fully represented by a rate of the cyclist body height, his body mass, as well as the inclination and length of his helmet. All the above mentioned factors have been thus taken into account in the modelling.

$$A = 0.045 \times h^{1.15} \times m_b^{0.2794} + \left[0.329 \times \left(L \times \sin\sin K_1\right)^2 - 0.137 \times \left(L \times \sin\sin K_1\right)\right]$$

where h is the height of the cyclist, m_b the body mass of the cyclist, L the length of the helmet, and α_1 the inclination of the head.

The prediction accuracy was then determined by comparisons between planimetry measurements and A values estimated using the model. Within the ranges of h, m_b, L and α_1 involved in the experiment, results have shown that the accuracy of the model is 3%. Within the objective to be easy to use, this accuracy can be considered sufficientenough to show the impact of postural and equipment changes on the value of the frontal area of cyclists. This model is explicit and it has been developed to take into consideration variation of posture i.e. inclination of the head. It can easily be applied to a variety of cyclists with different anthropometric characteristics since the height and body mass are input data. Moreover it can also considered the shape characteristic of the helmet including (L) its interaction with the inclination of the head (α_1). Finally its conditions of use are specified since its accuracy can only be guaranteed for input data that are within the ranges of h, m_b, L and α_1 involved in the experiment. It can thus provide pertinent indications useful for both coaches and cyclists.

On the Relevance of Aerodynamic Force Modelling vs. Wind Tunnel Testing

Individual and accurate optimization of the aerodynamic properties of athletes on very details modifications by means of wind tunnel measurements is essential for high performance. However, such comprehensive experiments in large scale wind tunnels lead to excessive measurement time and costs and require the disposability of athletes over unreasonably long periods. Even if accurate, wind tunnel tests have the disadvantage of not being able to be used anytime it is needed as it is required for high level sport. Moreover, the usual environmental conditions of the sport practice that can widely influence the performance are requirements that cannot be taken into account in a wind tunnel setting.

Instead, the computer modelling approach if well oriented allows studying the impact of all variables, parameters and initial conditions which determine the sport performance. In terms of aerodynamic, models implemented in the years 1980 and 1990, do not report the low dispersion of athletic performance neither because of the technical means available for their implementation nor because they were not designed for this purpose.

Several authors have tried to formalize the different steps to develop useful model but this process is not as linear as it seems. The first stage involves identifying the system under study. This is a situation analysis which will determine and describe the framework within which will take place all the work ahead. When the frame is set, it is about to implement procedures to collect data relating to the objective pursued. The choice of tools for collecting and processing experimental data must be consistent with the model and the desired accuracy. Wind tunnel testing can thus in this case be useful if it takes into consideration postures observed during training and racing, athlete/equipment interactions, boundary conditions. Then to build the model, dependencies between different recorded variables are considered. These relationships are then translated in the form of equations giving the model structure. According, it must be hierarchical and give the possibility to adapt to all levels of complexity, depending on the nature of the results to be obtained. Such models have an important value in the quest for performance if their results are express in term of objective benchmarks (time, speed, trajectories) that can extend the observation of the coaches.

They could have two exploitation level i.e. analytical or global since they enable stakeholders respectively to focus on a particular aspect of performance such as the specific influence of the aerodynamic resistance (analytical approach of the Newton's law) or on the interaction of factors determining the performance (global approach of the Newton's law)with the aerodynamic resistance among others. When such models are used for simulation, they allow stakeholders to go further than the simple description. Beyond the fact that they can be used anytime it is needed, they have also predictive capacities and that, at a lower cost.

Application and Valorisation: Towards an Optimization of Downhill Skiers' Performances when Passing Over a Bump

For each discipline in Alpine skiing (downhill, slalom, giant slalom), the difference in performance among the top world skiers is lower than one percent. Taking into account this low variability, coaches are confronted with the problem of assessing the efficiency of different postural strategies. Numerical models may provide an adequate solution. The method consists in computing a correlation between skiers' kinematics and postural parameters observed during training and each of the forces involved in the motion's equation. For postural strategies such as pre-jump or op-traken in downhill, models of the projected frontal area for the lift and for the drag are calculated based on postural parameters (length and direction of skier's segments).

$$A_L = 0.1167\sin(\vartheta) + 0.0258\sin(\beta) + 0.0607 + 0.024E_T((\sin\sin(2.\varpi_3) - \cos(\varpi_4))$$

Where A_L is the projected frontal area, is the orientation of the trunk, is the orientation of the tight in the sagittal plan, 3 and 4 are the arms orientation respectively in the frontal and horizontal plan.

$$A_D = 0.0003(L_1 \sin\sin(\mathrm{K}) + L_2 \sin\sin(\beta) + L_3 \sin\sin(\vartheta)) - 0.026 + 0.041(|\sin \varpi_1| + |\sin \varpi_2|)$$

Where A_D is the projected frontal area, is the orientation of the trunk, β is the orientation of the tight, α is the orientation of the shank in the saggital plan, $_1$ and $_2$ are both arms orientations in the horizontal plan.

Ground reaction and skis-snow friction are computed according to skiers' postural kinematics (skier's amplitude variation and duration of spread movements). Skiers' weight is easy to obtain. Thus the external forces exerted on the skis-skier system are known, the motion's equation can be solved and simulations performed. These can be used to estimate variations in time and loss in speed performance induced by different postural strategies.

Such simulations find an application in the field of training as they enable to assess the impact on performance of a given strategy compared with another. Simulation results can be presented in the form of animations, using DVD technology. Such tool enables trainers to show skiers very quickly the variability of performance induced by different postural strategies.

Broken down in this form, the simulation becomes a way of learning transmission. The aerodynamic drag model can be used directly, if the coach chooses to particularly focus his attention on the aerodynamic effects. A first level of use is then given to the model. Then the model can have a second level of use, if the coach wants to have a general view of the skier performance since it is also designed to be an integral part of the modeling of the postural strategies implemented by skiers when passing over a bump in downhill skiing.

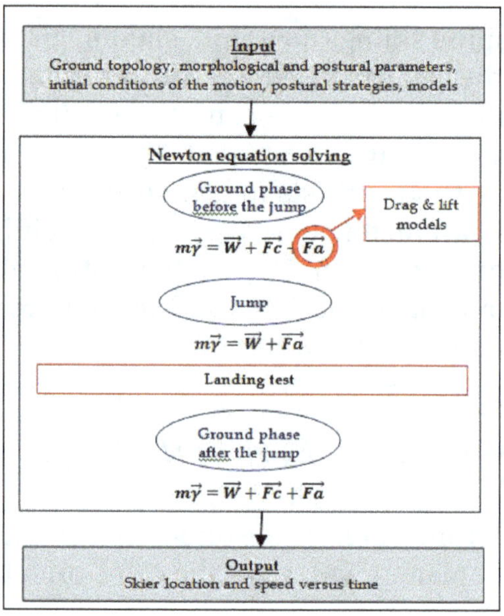

Structure overview of the simulator of the trajectory of the centre of mass of a skier according to his anthropometric characteristics and his postural strategy as well as the topology of the downhill slope.

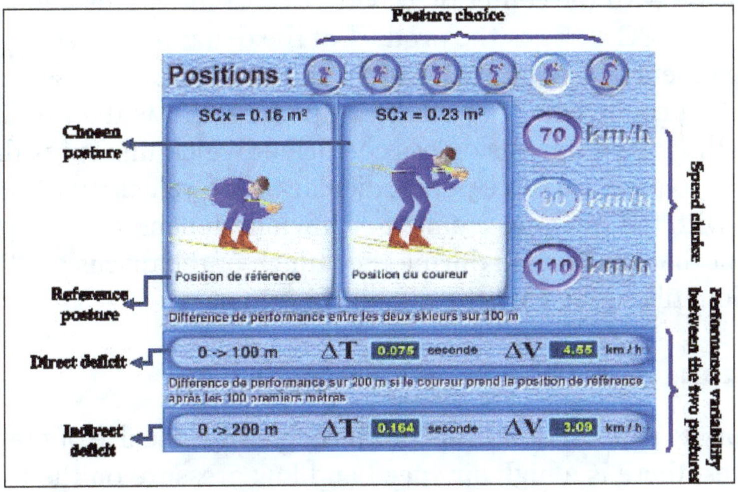

Overview of DVD application built for the downhill skiers of the French Ski Federation. The choice of a posture enables ones to see the aerodynamic drag impact on performance for three input speed. The choice of a particular input speed enables to see the aerodynamic drag impact according to six different postures usually observed during races. The direct performance variability in terms of time deficit and loss of speed between the reference posture and the chosen posture is given after 100 meters of straight running (Direct deficit). Then stakeholders can visualize the indirect deficit generate 100 meters further (200m) even if the skier adopt again an aerodynamic crouched posture (like the reference one) on the last 100 meters (Indirect deficit).

Aerodynamics of the Discus

The discus is an extremely aerodynamic implement. This implies that, under certain conditions, the distance thrown can be increased or decreased significantly beyond or below to that expected in a vacuum or in still air. A notable example is from the men's discus final during the 1976 Olympic Games, where the gold medalist released his discus a significant 1.4 m/sec., less than the silver medalist. However, aerodynamic factors dramatically affected the distance achieved by those two throwers. In a vacuum, the same author calculated that the silver medalist would have thrown 4.06 meters further than the winner. Indeed, the aerodynamic forces acting on the discus during its flight can decisively alter the course of its trajectory positively or negatively. So much so that the first author to publish scientific data regarding the effects of wind on the discus Taylor suggested that it would be unfair to allow records achieved under favorable conditions. Those favorable conditions are created as a result of fluctuations in the relative wind speed, primarily, and secondarily, the angle of release, the velocity of release, the attack angle, the inclination angle, the tilt angle, the rotation of the discus around its short and long axes, the effective mass of the discus and, its moment of inertia. During its flight the discus is influenced by gravity and the aerodynamic forces of lift, drag and pitching moment. Those forces act on the center of pressure (CP) which does not necessarily coincide with the center of gravity (CG) of the discus and is located somewhere in front of the CG. Drag is the product of the dynamic pressure (pressure in the front of the implement is greater than that in the rear), the cross-sectional area and a dimensionless drag coefficient. The other component, lift, is the product of the same elements but with its own dimensionless coefficient which measures the effectiveness of the implement to produce force perpendicular to the velocity vector. Those two coefficients along with the pitching moment coefficient depend on the attack angle. The angles of interest that are formed during the launch of the discus are those of release, attack, inclination, tilt, along with the pitching moment.

Lift Generation

The typical theory to explain how lift is produced, is with the use of the Bernoulli principle which states, there is a high air speed and low pressure on the top of the air foil (wing-discus-frisbee etc.) and a low speed and high pressure on the lower surface of the foil. The difference in pressure creates a positive, upward lift. However, this theory has been challenged as trivial, incorrect or incomplete (NASA). That is, it does not explain why the velocity is higher on top, and so the explanation of lift presented is no real explanation, or more precisely it is a trivial truism. Other theories that have been proposed include the Newton's third law theory, the "longer path" theory, the "downwash" theory, the Coanda effect theory, the Kutta-Zhukosky lift theory and the Prandtl Drag Theory. According to Johnson & Jansson none of these theories present a correct explanation of flight. They postulated that the aforementioned theories can be classified according to three conditions: trivial and correct, trivial and incorrect and, nontrivial but incorrect. They suggested that what is needed is a nontrivial correct theory and he offered a combination of the Bernoulli's principle and Newtonian physics theory as an explanation of how lift is generated. The detailed description of any of those theories is beyond the scope of this narrative.

Attack Angle

The optimum angle of attack of the discus depends on the angle of release. A negative angle of attack means that the initial direction of the center of gravity points upwards in relation to the long axis of the discus, with the opposite being true for a positive attack angle. Negative attack angles are the predominant in high level throwing. Generally, the negative angle of attack should increase as the angle of release increases and decrease as the angle of release decreases. At an approximate release angle of 25 degrees, the angle of attack is at zero. In still air, the optimized attack angle will be at -4 to -10 degrees. Along with other release parameters, Chiu, also calculated a -10.25° angle of attack as optimal for breaking the current men's world record, and that of -9.25° for breaking the current women's world record.

The magnitude of the lift, drag and pitching forces will strongly depend on the attack angle. According to Seo, Seo and Ganslen, lift increases linearly with the angle of attack up to the stalling angle which is at 30°. At that point the discus experiences a sudden decrease in lift and at 90° the lift force is zero. The drag force also increases with increasing attack angle from 0° to 90°. Ganslen showed that the sudden decrease in lift at 30° also coincides with the formation of a "turbulent wake" behind the discus. Discus performance will be improved if the discus has a relatively flat angle of attack. Once the discus develops an angle of attack to the relative wind, it will continue to exaggerate the "nose up" tendency which is termed as a positive pitching moment. This implies that a flight path initiated near the point of the stall angle for the discus, it will necessarily result in a stalled discus with high drag and low lift. Therefore, an optimum attack angle will allow the discus to complete its flight without stalling.

A term that has been used in reference to the attack angle, is the maximum lift/drag ratio and more specifically the attack angle at which that maximum ratio occurs. Taylor and Ganslen found that the maximum value of the ratio occurred at an attack angle of 9°. This value seems to be in conflict with a generally accepted negative optimal angle of attack. Hay attributed this discrepancy to the ever changing angle of attack during the discus's flight speculating that the optimum angle obtained at release will be the one that would yield the best results overall and not at a particular instant in flight. On the other hand Hubbard mentioned that the lift/drag ratio is a concept used in aircraft design to resolve issues related to the maximization of the steady cruising range of an aircraft. He stated that this ratio is irrelevant in a discussion of the transient behavior of a discus and that, as an aerodynamic term.

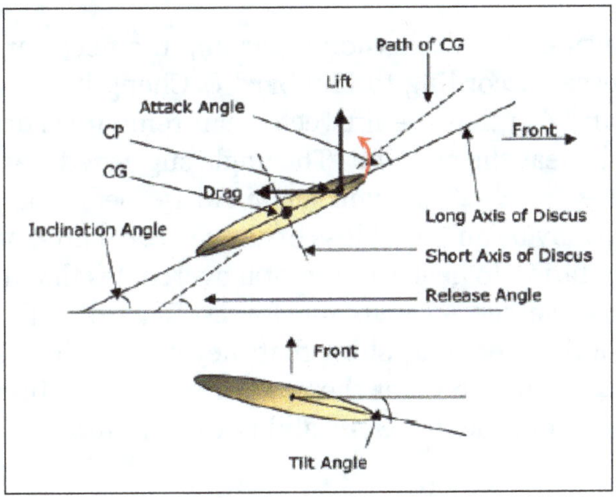

Release Angle, Angle of Tilt and Inclination Angle

Terauds reported that the angle of tilt at release should be at 15° which he probably estimated from field or film observations. Soong, found that with reasonable initial discus rotation, the release angle and the angle of inclination have a large effect on the range. At zero wind, the optimum combination of release angle and inclination angle is 35°/26° respectively if they vary independently. If they vary together, that optimum is at 33°. However, the former ratio will result in a 1.55 meters gain in range. Frohlich agreed that the optimum strategy in still air is to release the discus so that the inclination angle is about 5 to 10° less than the release angle. Although this results in negative lift during the early stages of the flight, it allows for a minimum of drag and optimum average lift throughout the upward part of the discus flight. Results from optimization studies that assumed a 0° angle of tilt, indicate that for elite throwers the discus should be thrown at release angles between 35-37°, inclination angles of 26-27°, and attack angles between -9 and -10°. Slightly higher release angles and more negative angles may be more suitable for throwers capable of lesser release speeds. Voigt claimed that by modifying his data to account for a -17° tilt angle at release, the range will improve by 2.7 meters. Hubbard & Cheng reported a maximum range of 69.39 meters with a men's discus released at windless conditions with a release speed of 25 m/sec. and a rotation of 6.6 rev/sec., is produced with an angle of release at 38.4°, inclination angle at 30.7°, and a tilt angle of 54.4° and attack angle at -4°. Deviations of several degrees of any of the first three values while holding the other Deviations of several degrees of any of the first three values while holding the other two constant, will result in a minimum decrease of the range achieved, i.e., less than 39 cm. Larger departures, in the order of tens of degrees, will result in a range decrease of approximately 5 meters. Generally, range is most sensitive to the release angle and least sensitive to the tilt angle at release. For both men's and women's discuses, the optimal initial conditions of the angles of release, inclination and tilt, will vary significantly with wind speed.

There has been a considerable discussion regarding the need for the presence or not of a tilt angle at release. According to Hubbard & Cheng it is optimal to release the discus tilted significantly so that the lift vector can remain vertical throughout much of the flight, especially near the end of it. The angle suggested was at 54.4°. That angle will gradually decrease, from 54° and will remain at 15° before landing for a nearly flat impact. Though there may be an initial loss of early vertical lift from that initial tilt, the eventual plane reorientation to nearly horizontal overcomes that disadvantage because the tilt results in larger average aerodynamic forces. Regarding the optimum tilt angle, casual observations of throwers may show that they release the discus with a tilt angle quite smaller than 54°. It may be that the application of a theoretical optimum angle may in the end detract from the throwers' ability to maximize release velocity or other release parameters.

Wind Velocity

It is a well established fact that for both men's and women's discuses, longer throws can be achieved throwing the discus against fairly strong winds than with the wind or no wind. The increases in range due to lift are larger than the decreases due to drag and the discus can always fly further in air than in vacuum. In an early investigation, Taylor, found that head winds between 7 and 8 mph were advantageous and that this advantage decreased progressively and at 14.5 mph became a disadvantage. He also found that tail winds of up to 14 mph were also detrimental to the range achieved. However, Frohlich using mathematical modeling, found that a discus will travel about 6 meters further if thrown in a 7.5 m/sec (16.8 mph) head wind than if thrown with the wind, and 8.2 meters further if thrown in a 20 m/sec (22.5 mph) headwind than with such wind. A properly thrown discus will always fly further if thrown against winds up to 20 m/sec (45 mph), than with it. This implies that long throws cannot be achieved against extremely strong winds. Theoretically, if the wind velocity is high enough, the discus will stop flying forward and it will actually travel backwards at some point during its flight.

Hubbard & Cheng, employing a 3D dynamic model, reported a 10 and 14 meters advantage for men and women when throwing into a 5 m/sec (11 mph) headwind compared to a 10 m/sec. (22 mph) tailwind. Tutjowitsch found that if thrown at an negative angle of attack and at a release speed of 23 m/sec, the discus will fly 5.4 meters further if thrown into a head wind of 5 m/sec (11 mph). This value is close to Taylor's but quite less that that of Frohlich. Unger claimed a linear increase in distance for head winds of up to 5 m/sec (11 mph) with a greater than linear relationship for higher wind speeds, although he provided no support for those claims.

Chiu, employing mathematical modeling, estimated optimal performances when the wind speed fluctuated from -21 m/sec (-47 mph) to 12 m/sec (27 mph). He found that when the head wind was at 17 m/sec (38 mph) the male "virtual" record holder could throw up to 84.27 meters, approximately 10 meters further than the current world record. When the head wind was over 17 m/sec., the range would decrease gradually. Similarly, for the female "virtual" record holder the distance would decrease at head wind speeds of over 13 m/sec (29 mph). Chiu also found that generally with increased tail wind, thrown distances for both males and females would decrease. However, he also reported a little known observation that, with tail winds of over 7 m/sec or 15.7 mph, the ranges thrown for both males and females would begin to increase adding about 2 meters in a throw of 72.28 m., when the tail wind increased to 12 m/sec., (27 mph). At that tail wind speed, the throwing distance would be the same as when throwing in windless conditions. Chiu also reported that when the head wind was approximately 8 m/sec. (18 mph), both male and female "virtual" record holders would obtain their optimal throwing distance provided that the angle of release and the inclination angle were the same. On the other hand, with increased tail wind the optimal distance could be obtained only when the inclination angle was larger than the release angle.

Regarding the drag and lift coefficients, Frohlich stated that the measurement of those is probably not accurate for relative wind speeds of over 40 m/sec (90 mph) and that it would not be meaningful to perform any range calculations with wind speeds above 20 m/sec (45 mph).

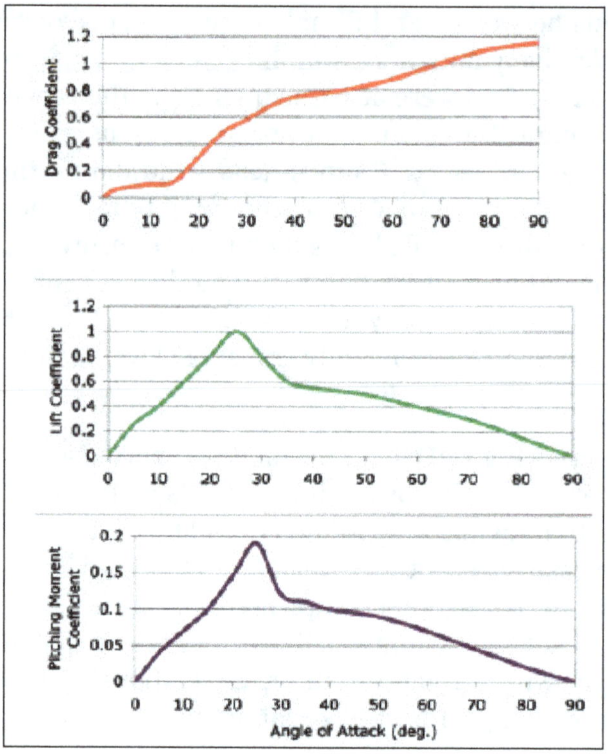

Throwing in the Wind

For moderate winds, i.e., less than 20 m/sec (45 mph), a discus thrown with a tail wind must be thrown with a different strategy than a discus thrown in a head wind. Frohlich stated that with a head wind, the discus inclination angle, at release, should be about 10° to 15° less than the release angle so that during the majority of the flight the drag will be kept at minimum and lift at maximum. As the velocity of the wind increases, the release angle decreases making the discus trajectory flatter. This way the discus will not hover for too long and stall towards the end of its flight. On the other hand, for a discus thrown into a tail wind, the release angle should increase, the discus is thrown higher in the air. With tail wind velocities over 20 m/sec (45 mph), longer throws will be obtained if the discus is turned over so the discus catches the wind like a sail would. The worst possible conditions to obtain long throws is to throw in a tail wind of 7.5 m/sec. (17 mph). If the wind velocity is less than about 20 m/sec. (45 mph), longer throws can always be achieved by throwing against the wind.

Frohlich also observed that although the longest throws take place against strong winds, it is easier to obtain optimum performances when throwing in a tail wind, in the sense that it is easier or, less technique demanding, for a thrower to produce the optimum release parameters than if throwing in a head wind. For example, to obtain a throw within one meter of the optimum when throwing in a 10 m/sec (22 mph) head wind, the thrower should release the discus at an angle within ±5° of the optimum and at a discus inclination angle within ±3° of the optimum. When throwing in a 10 m/sec (22 mph) tail wind, the thrower could release the discus within ±6°, and ±15° of those angles respectively, to come within the same one meter of the optimum throw. This may imply that throwing in head winds may favor the experienced thrower due to the larger control required to achieve optimum performances. In addition, the effect of a head wind is enhanced as the discus spin increases with the higher the spin, the better the effect of a headwind.

Hubbard & Cheng described what they termed a "slicing" strategy when throwing against strong headwinds of between 6 and 20 m/sec. (1345 mph). In those conditions it is optimal to initially have the discus symmetry plane (an imaginary plane that equally divides the discus front and back) nearly vertical by decreasing initial inclination and increasing initial tilt substantially (>70°), although the release angle remains relatively constant near 35°. With strong tailwinds very high release angles are optimal. For example, with tail winds at 10.8 m/sec (24 mph), a strategy of 44.3°, 36.7° and 58.6° (release angle, inclination angle, tilt angle) will produce the same result as a 46°, 46.3° and 19.1° strategy, other factors being equal. For large tailwinds, a "kiting" strategy was proposed taking advantage of the fact that in extreme conditions the wind speed may be greater that the discus horizontal velocity.

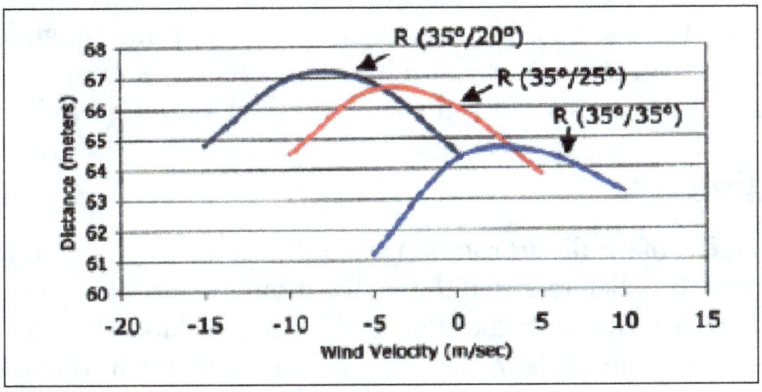

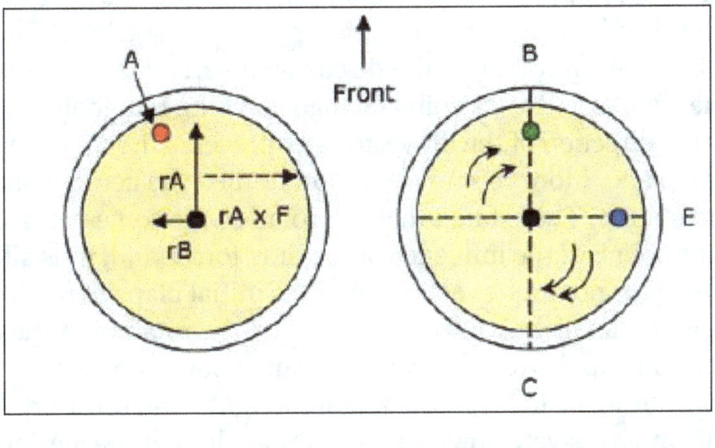

In this case an initially positive angle of attack is chosen which makes both the angle of release and the inclination angle to increase. For a tailwind of 20 m/sec (45 mph), an angle of release at 62° with an inclination angle at 90° is proposed, with the entire flight essentially occurring at that extreme inclination angle, and the discus acting like a sail. Obviously, those optimal theoretical angles for high winds are extremely difficult or impossible to obtain by throwers.

Ganslen mentioned that a less able thrower will benefit more from a head wind of a given speed than a good thrower, because the percentage increase in the relative wind will be greater for the less able thrower than a thrower who can throw the discus at high velocities. Soong, found that the head wind advantage is lost when the discus inclination angle is too high as it happens when both the angles of release and the inclination angle are 35°.

Realease Velocity

The paramount factor for optimum performance is the release velocity and all the efforts of the thrower should be geared towards enhancing that value. Aerodynamic forces become more important with increasing release velocity. Up to about 25 m/sec (56 mph), of release velocity, the range achieved is more or less the same whether the discus is thrown in windless conditions (still air) or in absolute vacuum, although a quite different angle of release should be used to obtain the optimal range for the throw. A discus will go further in still air as compared to a vacuum assuming that the release velocity is better than 25 m/sec., or if throwing against a strong wind.

Discus Rotation

The most salient effect of the discus rotation around its short axis, is to stabilize its orientation during its flight. Frohlich reported that at the moment of release, the discus rotates at approximately 7 rev/sec. However, the effect of the discus rotation had not been studied in all past investigations, many of them assuming that both the pitching and the rolling rates the of the discus are invariable due to the stabilization gyroscopic effect of the discus spin. Soodak and Hubbard and Cheng recognized the apparent characteristic of the discus flight to exhibit a slow but uneven rolling of the discus with several degrees of roll occurring in typical flights. The women's discus exhibits a higher rolling rate than the men's. This rolling motion alters the direction of the lift vector and prevents the trajectory from occurring in a purely vertical plane. More recently, Rouboa studied the aerodynamics of the discus with and without rotation. They stated that the rotation motion essentially influences the air resistance as it minimizes the influence of the drag forces and, thus allowing the discus to fly further. If there are no torques acting on it, the initial plane of motion of the discus is maintained throughout its flight. However, in reality, the rotation of the discus generates aerodynamic forces that apply torques which are small but not negligible. A careful observation of the discus during its flight shows that for a right hand thrower, the left side of the discus tilts or rolls progressively downwards at an angle that reaches approximately 10° shortly before the discus lands. This behavior of the discus occurs because the aerodynamic lift forces are larger on the forward half of the discus and tend to make the front edge move upwards. Because of the discus rotation, this upward torque creates a gyroscopic precession, a phenomenon occurring in rotating bodies in which an applied force is manifested 90 degrees later in the direction of rotation from where the force was applied. Therefore, the end result is the creation of a torque vector pointing to the right and causes the right side of the discus to go up. Secondly, since the discus rotation causes the relative air velocity to be slightly higher on the left side of the discus (Magnus effect), the aerodynamic forces cause a lateral displacement of the center of pressure to the left. These forces create a torque vector pointing forward causing the front edge of the discus to pitch upward at about 1.5°/sec during its flight which results in a change in the angle of attack which in turn affects the magnitude of the lift later in flight. Those three moment components (i.e., higher forces on the front half, lateral displacement of the center of pressure and, change in the attack angle) will rotate the discus counter clockwise around its long axis, with the left edge moving downwards and the front edge pitching up. It will also slow the rate of rotation of the discus around its own axis, although that effect is negligible. The latter authors also reported that optimal strategies and ranges for both men's and women's discuses depend on initial spin assuming a constant velocity and on release velocity assuming a constant spin. Frohlich mentioned that because of the symmetrical shape of the discus, a non rotating one would experience smaller aerodynamic torques than a rotating one and that this had caused an expert to suggest that a discus be constructed with a hollow rim filled with mercury in order to reduce that rotation after the release. However, a non-rotating discus lacks stability and will most likely wobble. Such a discus may experience less torque but it will also become less aerodynamic, and eventually the negative effects will outweigh the positive.

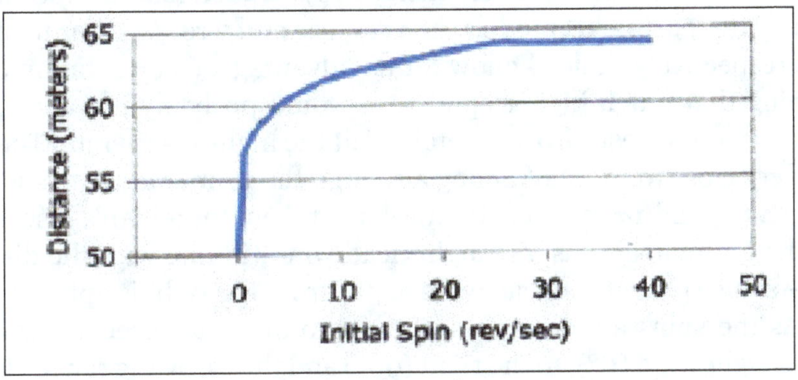

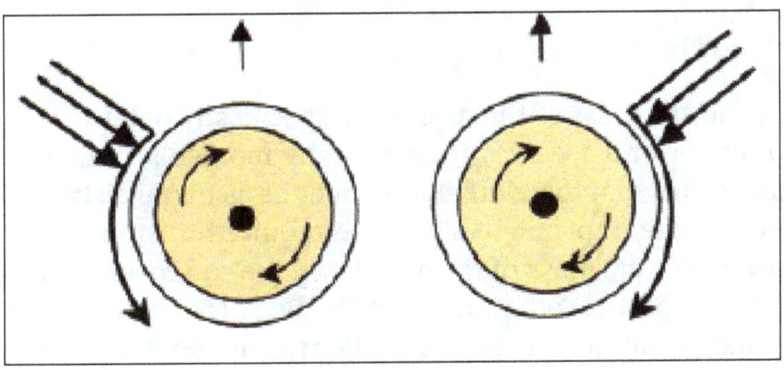

Rouboa, using computational fluid dynamics, studied the aerodynamic effects on the discus both with and without rotation. They found that the range of the discus was strongly affected by the drag coefficient, the initial velocity of release, the release angle and the direction of wind velocity. In turn, those variables change as a function of discus rotation. For a variety of angles of release and velocities of release they tested, the rotating discus had an advantage over the non rotating one. For example for release speeds of 25 m/sec (56 mph) and 27 m/ sec (60 mph), a rate of rotation at 4 rev/ sec, an angle of release at 34°, angles of attack varying between 0° and 90° and, a head wind of 10 m/sec (22 mph), there was a gain of the rotating discus of 2 meters and 5 meters respectively for those two release speeds. They also calculated that the rotation of the discus does not alter the vertical distance of the throw. However, those authors did not specifically mention whether the rotation of the discus affects drag, lift and pitch. Regarding that issue, Seo et al., found little difference between the aerodynamic coefficients of drag, lift and pitching moment whether the discus was spinning or not. Voigt reported a 3.75 meters increase in range if the spin was increased from 5 to 16 rev/sec. with a release speed of 20 m/ sec.

Soong also tested the effect of the speed of rotation of the discus. He found that with a 25.5 m/sec. speed of release and a discus rotation speed from 0 rev/ sec to 37 rev/ sec, there was an increase of 13.76 meters attributed to the discus rotation. Although he tested higher rotation speeds, he found out that values beyond the speed of approximately 37 rev/ sec., will not change the range achieved, but that the pitching and rolling motions could be reduced. Hubbard & Cheng, 2007, argued that the optimal initial spin rates they calculated, using 3D models, of 4 rev/sec and 7 rev/sec. for men's and women's discuses respectively, indeed allow for an advantageous orientation of lift later in flight something that much higher spin rates would probably not allow. Hildebrand similarly found that the best throw is obtained at the highest spin rate. Their numerical results were very close to those of Soong although the former authors studied rotation speeds between 6.3 and 14 rev/ sec. By the same token, for a men's discus spinning at 14 rev/sec., the optimal wind is a straight head wind (in line with the direction of the throw). At the same spin rate, a head wind at 50° from the right is optimal for the women's discus. As the spin rate decreases, the optimum wind direction generally shifts from a head straight wind (0°), to the right (90°) and the throwing range also decreases.

Moment of Inertia

The dimensions and the mass of the discus are specifically determined by the rules of the sport, but there are no specifics regarding the moments of inertia of the discus, which essentially means that there are no restrictions as to the distribution of the mass around the center of the implement. The force required to stop a rotating object depends on the product of the mass of the object and the square of the distance from the axis of rotation to the particles that make up the body (I= m r2). The further the distribution of the mass from the center, the greater the moment of inertia of the rotating object. Inertia simply expresses the degree of resistance in altering the given state of an object. Discuses with large moment of inertia have most of their weight towards the edge of the discus. Assuming that adequate rotation is imparted on such a discus, it will be increasingly difficult to alter its state of rotation, i.e., to slow it down. Indeed, most discus throwers have a tendency to prefer throwing discuses in which most of the mass is concentrated toward the rim. The large moment of inertia of those discuses, that resists changes, make them less prone to adverse aerodynamic torques. Since a discus with large moments of inertia is less likely to spin out of its previous rotational plane, the highest density of the discus should be on its circumference.

These days companies offer a plethora of discuses with a variety of weight distribution. The wise thrower will choose the discus that will suit her capabilities. More may not always be better when it comes to the moment of inertia of the discus. Soong studied the effect of the discus moment of inertia, as a function of the rate of discus spin, comparing two men's discuses, one with a 22.4 mm., rim thickness (most commonly used discuses) and another with 28.2 mm. The former presented inertia of 157.61 gm/cm/sec2, while the latter, 182.5 gm/cm/sec2. He found that the ratio of the moment of inertia to the weight of the commonly used discus, is already sufficiently high. Further effort in redistributing the mass will not produce significant improvement in the throw. The maximum distance advantage of the thicker rim discus was at the spin rate of 8 rev/sec., and it was about 44 cm, while at the speed of 4 rev/sec., the gain was 1 cm.

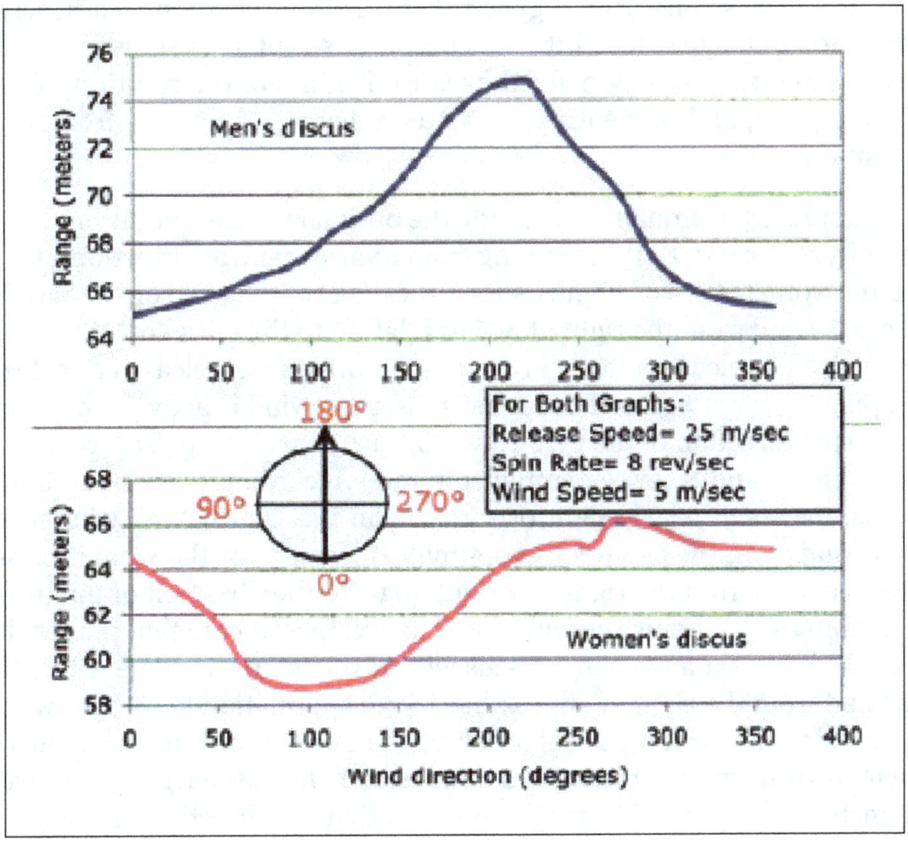

Other Effects

Side Winds: Simulation research has not extensively studied the effect of side winds. Experience with throwing against head side winds strongly supports the advantage of those winds. In an observation of a number of practice throws, Pharoah speculated that the optimum wind direction is from 20° to the right of the throwing direction. Frohlich also mentioned that head winds blowing from the right side (right hand throwers) would allow for even longer throws than those obtained with direct head-winds. He suggested that in those conditions the thrower would want to release the discus with the highest point of its rim towards the direction of the wind. He further explained that with the wind being from the right, it will reach the discus at oblique angles, and that the relative wind velocity will be smaller compared to a direct head-wind. This will cause both the drag and the lift to be reduced. However, longer distances may be obtained since some of the drag forces would act perpendicular to the direction of flight thus reducing their negative effect on the discus. In addition, Terauds has addressed that for a right hand thrower, the side wind from the right, would also serve to maintain the gyroscopic stability of the discus by enhancing the rotation of the discus since its right side moves with the wind rather than in opposition. For left hand throwers, the same phenomenon is true for a wind from the left and a counterclockwise rotation of the discus. Hildebrand further mentioned that with headwinds, the discus rolls from a generally horizontal position to a nearly vertical one which tends to make it lose lift. His computer simulation showed that the head wind from the right is more beneficial because it hinders the rotation of the discus around its long axis, and preventing, or better delaying, the discus from assuming a vertical position.

Hildebrand applied 3D simulation to study the optimal release conditions given a constant wind of 5 m/sec. (11.2 mph) blowing from a variety and all directions, for both the men's and the women's discus. Figure shows the effect of the wind on the range. For the men's discus, a wind from the right at 40° in relation to the direction of the throw, was the optimal, given a release velocity at 25 m/sec., an angle of release at 33 degrees and an initial spin at 8 rev/sec. For the women's discus, a wind exactly from the right, 90° in relation to the direction of the throw, was optimal, given 24 m/sec. release velocity, 41° angle of release and 8 rev/sec initial spin rate. According to those authors, for the men's discus, the result is a straightforward one in that a direct tail wind is the worst and a head wind from the right is the optimal. However, for the women's discus, the optimal wind comes from the right at a right angle to the direction of the throw (90°), with winds from the left being the worst. It is interesting to note that the results of Hildebrand et al. show that a women's discus will travel about the same with a direct tail wind or a wind from the right at approximately 30° in relation to the throw, assuming all other variables are constant. Also, based on the same results, for the men's discus, a thrower who is throwing the discus in a wind exactly from the right (90°), would gain about 1.2 meters if he adjusted his technique so that the direction of the discus flight shifts about 15° to the right.

Effects of Discus Area, Mass, Air Density: The effect of the aerodynamic forces is proportional to the quantity Area/Mass. In those quantities, the mass and area of the discus are fixed values, whereas the air density can fluctuate among places depending on temperature and altitude. Frohlich reported that, assuming same release velocity, lower effective mass discuses fly further, particularly in a head wind. In still air, for every kilo in mass reduction there are 47 cm. gain in distance, whereas in a headwind of 10 m/sec., (22 mph) the gain in distance is approximately 3 meters for every kilo in mass reduction. This implies that, if released at the same velocity, a women's discus will travel 47 cm. further than the men's in still air and 3 meters further in a headwind of 10 m/sec., due to the better overall aerodynamics of the reduced surface women's discus. When the effective mass is reduced, the thrower will need to reduce the release angle to obtain the optimum distance. Therefore, women discus throwers should release their discus several degrees smaller than the suggested optimum for the men's discus. Men discus throwers throwing at high temperatures and high altitudes should release at angles several degrees beyond suggested optimal. Hildebrand et al. also attributed differences between the men's and women's discuses, as to the optimal direction of the wind, to differences in the discus effective mass.

Effects of Gravity, Orientation and Release Height: Because the gravitational acceleration varies less than 0.5 percent among places on Earth, changes in that acceleration have little effect on discus range, a discus will fly 34 cm. farther at the equator than at the poles. Moreover, because of the earth's rotation, any projectile will travel longer if released eastward than westward, assuming no differences in any of the other factors affecting the distance thrown. The distances gained will be minimal though.

Regarding the release height, Frohlich reported that it appears that releasing the discus 1 meter higher will result in a 2 meter longer range. Since such increases in release height are impractical, those gains can be generalized and assumed to be approximately 10 cm for every 5 cm increase in release height.

Aerodynamics of the Javelin

Javelin throwing is a highly technical event and requires perfect coordination of multiple joints in different planes of motion.

The distance a javelin is thrown is affected by factors such as wind speed and direction and the aerodynamics of the javelin. But the two most important and controllable factors are javelin release speed and release angle.

Three steps to a speedy release:

1. Run up and crossover steps: a javelin throw involves a run-up of six to 10 steps, followed by two or three crossover steps before the thrower releases the javelin.

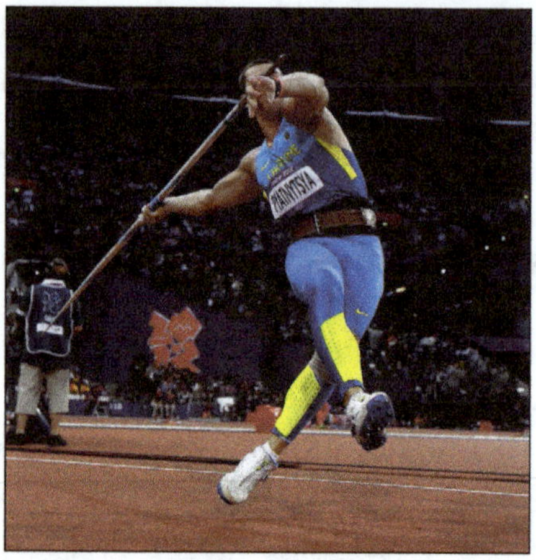

Crossover steps.

The first running steps are used to build the speed and rhythm of the thrower. The thrower then moves into crossover steps facing the side. These allow the thrower to continue to increase speed while setting up for an good release position.

The average maximum run up speed of an elite thrower ranges from 5-6m/s (20km/h), but elite throwers release the javelin at 28-30m/s (100km/h) so most of the final release speed is created in the "whole body" action of the final two steps.

The second-last crossover step, known as the impulse step, is slightly exaggerated to allow the thrower to land with their weight over their back foot, a similar movement to a cricket fast bowler. It makes sure the thrower is in the right position to start the throwing motion.

2. Transfer: The final step, known as the delivery step, allows the thrower to transfer the momentum built from the run up into the javelin. This is achieved in a movement that moves from the centre of the throwers body to the end of the throwers limbs. It is a whip-like transfer of energy from the hip to shoulder to elbow to javelin.

The delivery begins as the thrower lands on their back foot with a long straight arm and the javelin tip in line with their eyes.

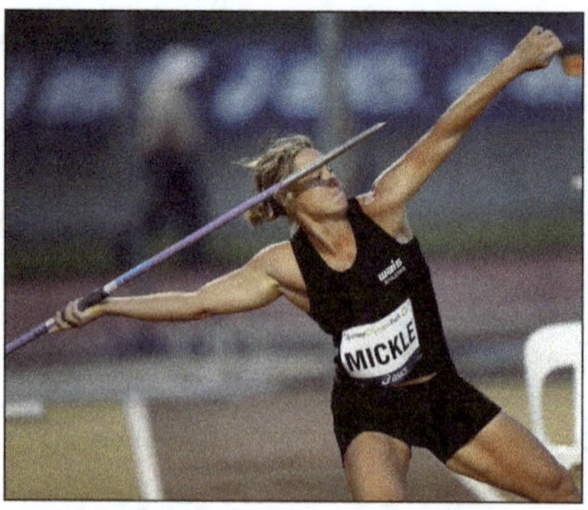

The first movement is to begin rotating the right knee and right hip while maintaining the position of the upper body.

The front foot is planted with a braced straight leg with the aim of "blocking" and minimising the bend of the knee, so that the thrower's right side quickly moves around the left.

A force six to eight times the athlete's body weight is created at front foot contact. A bent or "soft" knee will result in a loss of energy transfer, so it's important for javelin throwers to develop the leg and ankle strength to handle these large forces.

3. Delivery and recovery: Once the front foot is down, the motion of the upper body begins. As one joint – such as the hip – reaches the end of its range of motion and decelerates, the next joint – the shoulder, then elbow and finally the javelin – is rapidly accelerated.

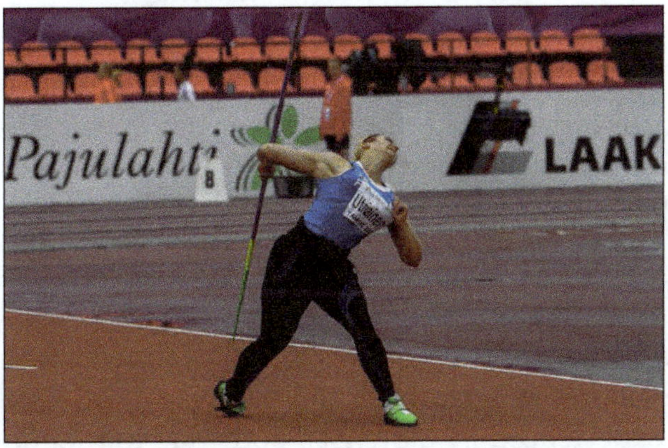

The final result is a high release speed on the javelin itself.

The javelin is thrown over the top of the shoulder with a bend in the thrower's side, similar to a fast bowler. But javelin throwers, unlike fast bowlers, are required to come to a complete stop before the foul line within one or two steps of release, creating a huge amount of stress on lower body joints.

Angle of Release

The second important parameter is the angle at which the javelin is thrown. The best angle of release for a javelin is between 32° and 36°, but this is tough to achieve consistently.

The flight path and distance of the javelin depends on the angle of attack, which is the difference between the:

- Angle of attitude: The orientation of the javelin to the ground.
- Angle of velocity vector: The flight path of the javelin's centre of mass (not the tip).

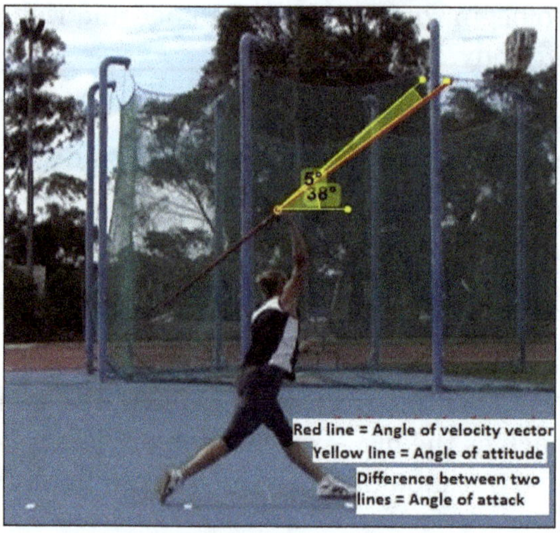
5°
38°
Red line = Angle of velocity vector
Yellow line = Angle of attitude
Difference between two lines = Angle of attack

Javelin release angle definitions.

The ideal angle of attack is zero degrees.

If the angle of attitude is larger than the angle of velocity vector, the javelin won't travel in the most aerodynamic way. Its increased surface area will slow it down and decrease the throw length, especially in a headwind.

Aerodynamic Factors in Cycling

In order to better understand the aerodynamics of cycling, it is important to first understand how air resistance is calculated. Below is the drag equation that represents the drag force, F_D, experienced by a cyclist's body due to the movement through the air. The first element of the equation is the density of the air, ρ, which decreases with altitude, thus one way to experience less drag is to move from the sea level to the mountains.

The second factor is A, the projected frontal area of the cyclist on a bike. In general, the smaller the frontal area, the smaller the drag—thus in order to minimize air resistance, the cyclists have to make themselves as small as possible on the bike. The next component—the drag coefficient C_D—depends on a number of factors including speed and surface roughness, and it has to be measured directly. Finally, $\mathbf{v}$, the cyclist's velocity relative to the air around them plays a role. The velocity is squared, which means the cyclist that goes twice as fast experiences four times the drag.

$$F_D = \frac{1}{2}\rho A C_{D^{V}}{}^{2}$$

Aerodynamics of Cycling Visualized

The airflow around a cyclist in three different positions was simulated. The first is an upright position with the hands on top of the handlebars. Here most of the cyclist's torso is presented to the wind, so it is not expected to be a very aerodynamic position. The second position puts the rider's hands lower on the handlebars in what cyclists call the "drops"—it leans the rider further forward and is a typical racing position both on flat terrain and on the descent. The last position has the rider crouched even lower, on the bike's top tube—it's extremely hard to pedal in this position so it's only used when riding downhill.

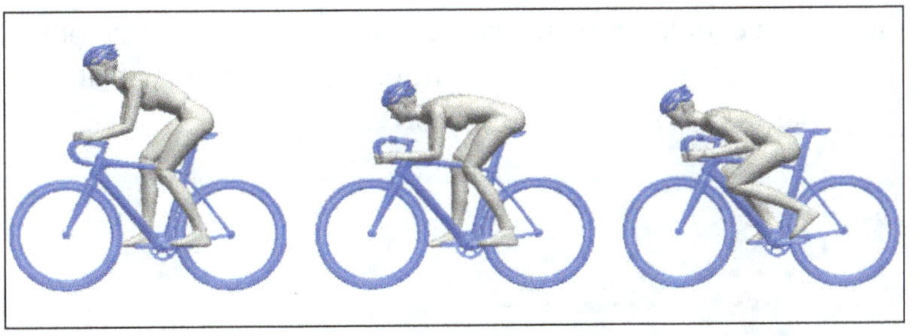

The three positions vary greatly in the frontal area A—the "drops" and top bar positions are 20% and 34% smaller than the upright position. The simulation was performed with the conditions of 50 km/h at sea level, and the drag in the second and third positions was 14% and 32% lower respectively—so by making themselves smaller on a bike, cyclists cannot reduce the drag by an equal amount.

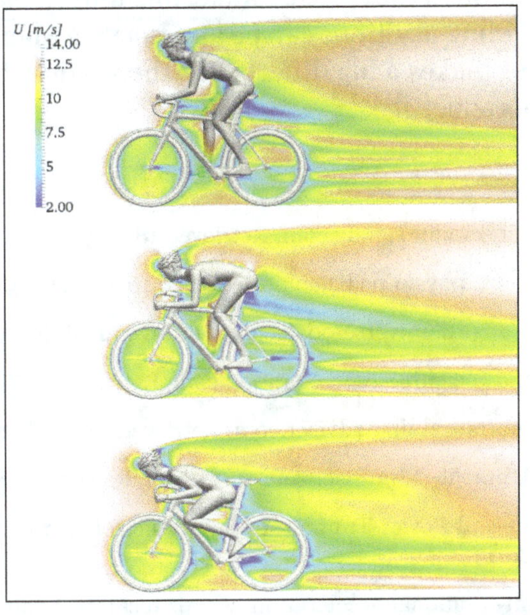

To understand why, consider the airflow around the three cyclists. The simulation image on the left shows air velocity around the cyclists. Notice that there is a large region of slower velocity right behind the saddle, especially in the case of the upright cyclist, which indicates a lot of drag. By getting lower on the bike, the cyclist is able to shrink the extent of this slow-moving region, but can never get rid of it completely, even in the top tube position.

The 3D structure indicates an association between the different parts of the flow with the areas on the cyclist—for example, the slower area associated with the cyclist's head, which fades as they move away. There is also a distinctive asymmetry to the cyclist's wake—it comes from the way the air flows around the cyclist's torso and legs, so it would change with the leg position as the cyclist pedals.

Other positions demonstrate some distinctive differences. In the "drops" position, the helmet area fades more quickly and we see a little less asymmetry behind the cyclist's body. With the cyclist crouched on the top tube, the region of the slower air gets compressed and the cyclist is overall much more streamlined.

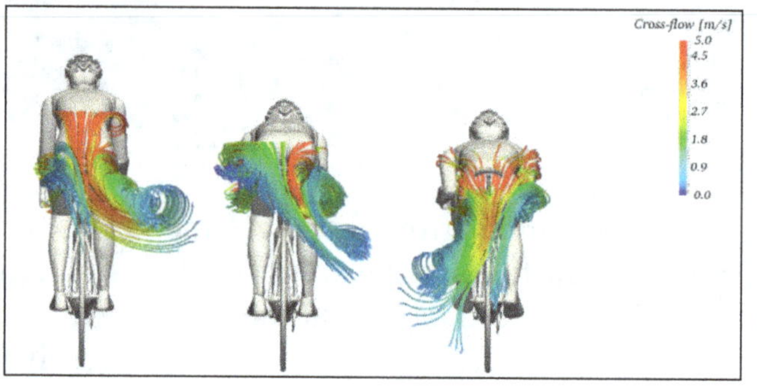

To get a sense of the rotation in the cyclist's wake, one must look at the streamlines. The difference between the riding positions can be appreciated when seen from behind. It is shown that getting lower makes a big difference—the vortices become smaller and the cross-flow velocities are reduced.

References

- Kinematics-of-human-motion: study.com, Retrieved 18 May, 2019
- Biomechanics-In-Sport: physio-pedia.com, Retrieved 16 June, 2019
- Gravitational-force- 75321: universetoday.com, Retrieved 18 July, 2019
- Gravity-speeds-friend-foe: athletesacceleration.com, Retrieved 17 May, 2019
- Principlesofforce: sports-training-adviser.com, Retrieved 16 April, 2019
- Rate-of-force-development-rfd-2: scienceforsport.com, Retrieved 08 August, 2019
- Transfer-of-Strength-and-Power-Training-to-Sports-Performance- 23711951: researchgate.net, Retrieved 19 June, 2019
- Angular-acceleration-rotational-acceleration: whatis.techtarget.com, Retrieved 14 May, 2019
- Sport-aerodynamics-on-the-relevance-of-aerodynamic-force-modelling-versus-wind-tunnel-testing, wind-tunnels-and-experimental-fluid-dynamics-research: intechopen.com, Retrieved 20 June, 2019

4

Nutrition for Sport and Exercise

Nutrition is important for athletes to maintain the daily intake of essential nutrients. Sports nutrition is a field that aims to understand the need and impact of proper nutrition in athletes. This chapter delves into diverse aspects of nutrition with respect to sport and exercise such as supplements, multivitamins and various other energy sources.

Sports Nutrition

Sports nutrition is a specialization within the field of nutrition that partners closely with the study of the human body and exercise science. Sports nutrition can be defined as the application of nutrition knowledge to a practical daily eating plan focused on providing the fuel for physical activity, facilitating the repair and rebuilding process following hard physical work, and optimizing athletic performance in competitive events, while also promoting overall health and wellness. The area of sports nutrition is often thought to be reserved only for "athletes," which insinuates the inclusion of only those individuals who are performing at the elite level. The term athlete refers to any individual who is regularly active, ranging from the fitness enthusiast to the competitive amateur or professional. Differences may exist in specific nutrient needs along this designated spectrum of athletes, creating the exciting challenge of individualizing sports nutrition plans.

To fully understand and subsequently apply sports nutrition concepts, professionals instructing athletes on proper eating strategies first need to have a command of general nutrition as well as exercise science. The second step is to gain the knowledge of how nutrition and exercise science are intertwined, understanding that physical training and dietary habits are reliant on each other to produce optimal performance. The final step can be considered one of the most critical—the practical application of sports nutrition knowledge to individual athletes participating in a sport or physical activity.

Sports nutrition professionals must be able to teach athletes by putting "book" knowledge into practice with actual food selection and meal planning, while keeping in mind the challenges presented by busy schedules of exercise, competitions, work, school, and other commitments. It is this third step that many professionals lack after graduating from an undergraduate or graduate program in sports nutrition, dietetics, exercise science, or athletic training.

Basic Nutrients

Foods and beverages are composed of six nutrients that are vital to the human body for producing energy, contributing to the growth and development of tissues, regulating body processes, and preventing deficiency and degenerative diseases. The six nutrients are carbohydrates, proteins, fats, vitamins, minerals, and water and are classified as essential nutrients. The body requires these nutrients to function properly; however, the body is unable to endogenously manufacture them in the quantities needed daily, and therefore these nutrients must be obtained from the diet. Carbohydrates, proteins, and fats are classified as macronutrients because they have a caloric value and the body needs a large quantity of them on a daily basis. The micronutrients include vitamins and minerals; the prefix micro is used because the body's daily requirements for these nutrients are small. Water fits into its own class, and requirements for it vary greatly among individuals.

Carbohydrates

Carbohydrates are compounds constructed of carbon, hydrogen, and oxygen molecules. Carbohydrates are converted into glucose in the body, providing the main source of fuel (4 calories per gram of carbohydrate) for all physical activity. Carbohydrates are found in a wide variety of foods, including grains, fruits, and vegetables, as well as in the milk/alternative (soy, rice, nut, and other nondairy products) group.

Proteins

Amino acids are the building blocks of proteins, which are constructed of carbon, hydrogen, oxygen, and nitrogen molecules. Amino acids can be made within the body (nonessential) or obtained from dietary sources. Proteins are involved in the development, growth, and repair of muscle and other bodily tissues and are therefore critical for recovery from intense physical training. Proteins ensure that the body stays healthy and continues working efficiently by aiding in many bodily processes. Protein can also be used for energy, providing 4 calories per gram; however, it is not used efficiently and therefore is not a source of energy preferred by the body. Proteins are found in a variety of foods, including grains and vegetables, but are mainly concentrated in the milk/alternative as well as meat and beans/alternative (soy products, nuts, seeds, beans, and other nonanimal products) groups.

Fats

Fats, like the other macronutrients, are compounds made up of carbon, hydrogen, and oxygen molecules. Fats are also known as lipids, and they come from both plant and animal sources in our diet. Triglycerides are the most common type of fat. Other fats include cholesterol and phospholipids. With 9 calories per gram, fats are a concentrated source of energy. Fat is primarily used as a fuel at rest and during low to moderate-intensity exercise. Fats are also involved in providing structure to cell membranes, aiding in the production of hormones, forming the insulation that wraps nerve cells, and facilitating the absorption of fat-soluble vitamins. Fats are concentrated in butter, margarines, salad dressings, and oils, but they are also found in meats, dairy products, nuts, seeds, olives, avocados, and some grain products.

Vitamins

Vitamins are a large class of nutrients that contain carbon and hydrogen, as well as possibly oxygen, nitrogen, and other elements. There are two main requirements for a substance to be classified as a vitamin. First, the substance must be consumed exogenously because the body cannot produce it or cannot produce it in sufficient quantities to meet its needs. Second, the substance must be essential to at least one vital chemical reaction or process in the human body. Vitamins do not directly provide energy to the body; however, some vitamins aid in the extraction of energy from macronutrients. Vitamins are involved in a wide variety of bodily functions and processes that help to keep the body healthy and disease free. Vitamins are classified as either water soluble (B vitamins and vitamin C) or fat soluble (vitamins A, D, E, and K), depending on their method of absorption, transport, and storage in the body. Vitamins are found in nearly all foods, including fruits, vegetables, grains, meat and beans/alternative, milk/alternative, and some fats.

Minerals

Minerals are also a large group of nutrients. They are composed of a variety of elements; however, they lack carbon. Minerals have a role in the structural development of tissues as well as the regulation of bodily processes. Physical activity places demands on muscles and bones, increases the need for oxygen-carrying compounds in the blood, and increases the loss of sweat and electrolytes from the body, all of which hinge on the adequate intake and replacement of dietary minerals. Minerals are categorized into major minerals (calcium, sodium, potassium, chloride, phosphorus, magnesium, and sulfur) and trace minerals (iron, zinc, copper, selenium, iodine, fluoride, molybdenum, and manganese) based on the total quantity required by the body on a daily basis. Similar to vitamins, minerals are found in a wide variety of foods, but mainly are concentrated in the meat and beans/alternative and milk/alternative groups.

Water

Forming a category of its own, water deserves to be highlighted because of its vital roles within the body. The human body can survive for a much greater length of time without any of the macro- or micronutrients than without water. The body is 55–60% water, representing a nearly ubiquitous presence in bodily tissues and fluids. In athletics, water is important for temperature regulation, lubrication of joints, and the transport of nutrients to active tissues. In addition to plain water, water can be obtained from juices, milk, coffee, tea, and other beverages, as well as watery foods such as fruits, vegetables, and soups.

How does the Body Produce Energy?

The body derives its energy from foods ingested daily. Carbohydrates, fats, and proteins are known as the energy nutrients because they serve as the body's source for energy. These energy nutrients are quite literally chemicals that have energy trapped within the bonds between the atoms of which they are made. The energy trapped within these nutrients is released when metabolic pathways within the cells break down the foods into their constituent parts, carbon dioxide and water. Some of the energy released is conserved or captured and used to make another high-energy chemical called adenosine triphosphate (ATP). The rest of the energy is lost as heat. ATP is the body's direct source of energy for cellular work. Without a constant source of ATP, muscles would not be able to generate force, and thus athletes would not be able to move or perform any physical activity.

Dietary Assessment Methods for the Athlete

Investigating what an athlete eats is a daily activity for a sports dietitian, so it would be expected that the practice would make it an efficient and effective task. However, dietary assessment remains a challenge in sports nutrition, with the potential for significant errors of validity and reliability. These errors challenge the accuracy of estimates of what the athlete actually ate, or usually eats, and may also prevent the detection of a real change if an assessment is repeated. Developing expertise in this activity requires an appreciation that there are different reasons for undertaking an assessment, different approaches to completing it and different tools that can be employed. Therefore, the outcome can be enhanced by matching the best approach to each specific situation. Nevertheless, there is also a need to take into account the errors involved in a dietary assessment when interpreting the data that is collected.

Reasons for Collecting Dietary Information

Two basic scenarios explain why athletes might want to collect information about their food intake. In the first, the interest is in measuring what an athlete actually eats during a period in which they make their own choices. The chief goal of this activity, typically termed a dietary assessment, is to investigate what is happening without influencing the process. This scenario occurs in sports nutrition in a variety of situations of both research and athlete servicing, each with its own challenges and specific goals Generally, dietary assessment methods are divided into strategies that are retrospective (what the athlete ate in the past) and those that are prospective (what happens over a period in the future). There have been four main methods used over the past 50 yrs to assess the dietary practices of athletes.

The second scenario, often known as diet tracking or self-monitoring, takes advantage of a limitation of many dietary assessment methods – that an individual will change his or her food intake during the process of monitoring it. A key tool in assisting an athlete to alter his or her dietary practices is to increase their self-awareness of their behaviour and the factors that underpin it. An athlete is likely to improve their food choices and portion control when they are accounting for their actions in real-time or directly associating their behaviour with an outcome. Receiving positive feedback about improvements in dietary practices and identifying the factors that support it can be valuable strategies in consolidating new habits.

Retrospective Measurements of Dietary Intake

Retrospective methods include the dietary history (a guided interview usually used to gain insights on habitual intake, often framed as a typical day), the 24 h recall (which investigates intake over a specific day) and the food frequency questionnaire (a summary of usual intake of different categories of foods). A general principle common to each of these techniques is that they are heavily reliant on the athlete's ability to recall the types and quantities of foods and drinks consumed over the period of interest in the past. These methods fall short when the athlete is embarrassed/unwilling to reveal his/her true eating patterns or unable to provide good descriptions of the type and amount of items in his/her past intake. The 24 h recall is the least frequently used protocol, because situations in athlete practice or research in which we are only concerned about what happened on a single day are not as common as other interests. Food frequency questionnaires and dietary histories generally attempt to assess intake over longer periods of time, which is valuable in gaining a longer-term perspective on eating patterns. However, these techniques are reliant on the athlete's memory and insights into their true intake and suffer when the athlete is a poor historian and/or has a complicated lifestyle that is difficult to summarize.

The dietary history is commonly used by sports dietitians to gain initial insight into an athlete's dietary practices. Although it does not lend itself to an accurate quantitative assessment of nutrient intake, it is valuable for gaining insight into the pattern of meals, snacks, intake around training sessions/events and supplement use. It requires a skillful interview technique to gather information with minimal bias, to cross-check the information, and to probe for factors that contribute to the patterns of intake. Although it is challenged by the athlete's ability to accurately describe the usual portion sizes of their food and drink choices, the use of models or pictures of food sizes can assist the athlete to better describe the quantities they consume.

Food frequency questionnaires (FFQ) can be implemented by a trained interviewer, but can also be self-administered by the athlete, using paper or an electronic format, to save time and resources. Asking athletes to identify how often they eat a range of individual food/drink items may gain a summary of the total diet, but tends to overestimate intake in low-energy consumers and under-estimate intake in large eaters. Importantly, it strips away some of the information that sports dietitians are interested in – for example, when a food or drink is consumed and what else is consumed at the same time. Food frequency questionnaires are most useful to assess the intake of a particular nutrient or food factor of interest – e.g., antioxidants or calcium – where, ideally, the FFQ has been validated by comparing responses to a biomarker of the intake or nutritional status of the compound. Again, models or pictures of foods and portion sizes can help to enhance the accuracy of the identification or quantification of dietary intake.

Fuels for Exercise

Fat and carbohydrate (CHO) provide the vast majority of fuel required for energy production in skeletal muscle during all intensities of aerobic exercise in humans. CHO also is consumed during 'anaerobic' (oxygen independent) exercise to sustain work rates performed above an individual's maximal aerobic power (VO2 max). CHO is available within the muscle fibre (in the form of glycogen) and from blood glucose (from the breakdown of liver glycogen). Fat is available from triglyceride (TG) droplets within the muscle fibre (intramuscular triglyceride, IMTG) as well as from plasma free fatty acids (FFAs) from lipolysis.

The glycogen content of skeletal muscle of untrained individuals consuming a mixed diet is typically 80 mmol/kg of muscle wet weight (ww). For individuals involved in regular strenuous endurance training, muscle glycogen content is somewhat higher at approximately 125 mmol/kg ww. After several days of a high (8–10 g/kg body mass) CHO diet and a decrease in training, muscle glycogen content can be elevated to values greater than 200 mmol/kg ww. As 1 g of glycogen is stored in tissue with 2 to 3 g of water, an athlete may have a 2 to 3% increase in body mass after several days of CHO loading. In addition to skeletal muscle reserves, about 100 g of glycogen are stored in the liver: liver glycogen can be hydrolysed back to glucose and transported via the bloodstream to working muscle for oxidation.

Adipose tissue TG constitutes by far the largest energy store in the body, sufficient to sustain skeletal muscle contraction for approximately 120 hours at marathon running pace! On the other hand, if only CHO were utilised as a fuel, it would deliver energy for approximately only 90 minutes of running. As the men's world record for the marathon is approximately 125 minutes, this highlights the importance of fuel integration during prolonged exercise. The size of the adipose tissue TG pool is difficult to estimate and obviously depends on the fat mass of each individual, but is likely to range from 50 000 to 100 000 kcal (approximately 200 000 to 420 000 kJ) in men and women with 10 to 30% body fat. In order for this TG to be used as a substrate for oxidative metabolism, it has to be exported from adipose tissue and transported by the blood to the active tissues where it will be utilised.

An important physiological store of fat is IMTG, stored adjacent to the mitochondria: the total active muscle mass may contain up to 300 g of IMTG within the myocyte as small lipid droplets, although this amount can vary substantially due to individual differences in fibre type (type I fibres contain a greater concentration of IMTG than type II fibres), endurance training status, and diet. Paradoxically, although regular endurance training elicits an increase in IMTG concentration in healthy individuals, an adaptation viewed as beneficial for training and performance, IMTG stores are also increased in patients with type 1 diabetes mellitus. This latter condition is associated with the features of insulin resistance syndrome.

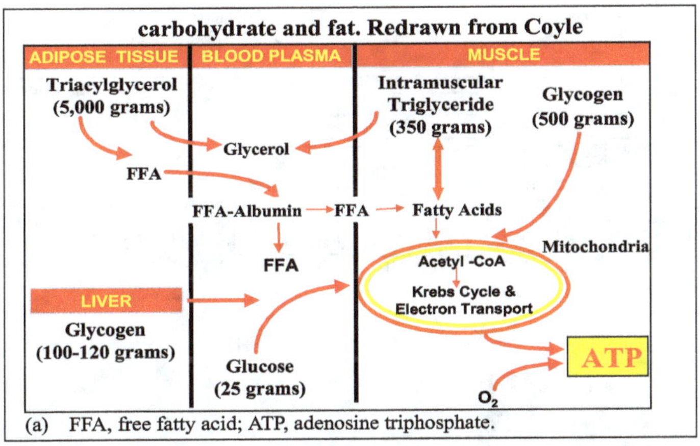

A schema of the major endogenous storage sites of carbohydrate and fat. Redrawn from Coyle.

Finally, fatty acids also can be derived from circulating TG (chylomicrons) and very low density lipoproteins (VLDL) formed from dietary fat in the post-absorptive state. Recent evidence suggests that if all the circulating VLDL-TG were taken up and oxidised, VLDL-TG degradation could contribute up to 50% of the lipid oxidised during sub-maximal exercise.

As an energy source, fatty acids have several advantages over CHO: The energy density of lipid is higher (37.5 kJ/g for stearic acid versus 16.9 kJ/g for glucose), while the relative weight as stored energy is lower. Fatty acids also provide more adenosine triphosphate (ATP) per molecule than glucose (147 versus 38 ATP), although the complete oxidation of fatty acid requires more oxygen than the oxidation of CHO (6 versus 26 mol of oxygen per mole of substrate for glucose and stearic acid oxidation, respectively). However, despite the vast stores of endogenous TG, the capacity for fatty acid oxidation during exercise is limited. Unlike CHO oxidation, which is closely geared to the energy requirements of the working muscle, there are no mechanisms for matching the availability and utilisation of fatty acid to the rate of energy expenditure. As a result, the rate of fatty acid oxidation during aerobic exercise is largely determined by the availability of fatty acid, the rate of CHO utilisation and the exercise intensity.

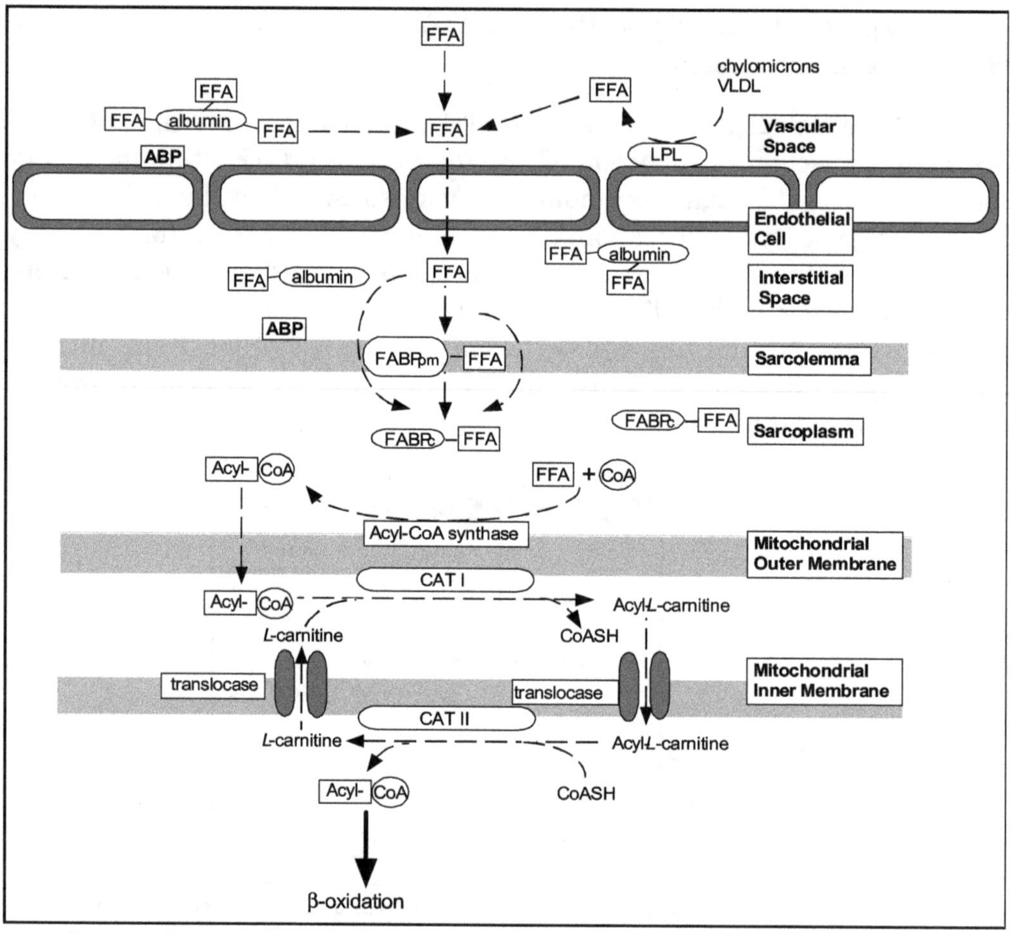

A schema of the transport of fatty acids from the vascular space to the inner mitochondria of the skeletal muscle where ß-oxidations occurs.

There are many potential sites at which the ultimate control of fatty acid oxidation may reside, with the relative importance of each site depending on a myriad of external factors such as the aerobic training status of the individual, habitual dietary intake, ingestion of substrates (CHO and fat) before and during exercise, gender, and the relative and absolute exercise intensity.

Energy Bar

Sports nutrition concentrates on athletic performance. It plays important role in keeping athletes healthy, preventing fatigues and illness associated with poor recovery.

The various varieties of bars available in the global market with good organoleptic properties. These bars are generally packed in metallised polyester films and have a limited shelf life of 3 to 4 months.

Energy bars are a dietary supplement often consumed by athletes and other physically active people to maintain their Calorific needs. Energy bars provide the strength and vitality for sustained physical and mental activity. It is meant to be high in carbohydrates and moderate protein content.

The purpose of the energy bar is to provide energy conveniently and quickly during endurance training or any kind of sports or exercising events. A Typical energy bar weighs between 45g to 80g and is likely to supply about 200-300 kcals; 7-15g of protein; 3-9g of fat and 20-40g of carbohydrates.

People concerned in getting healthier and keeping the good body fitness such as sporting and exercising individuals have changed their eating patterns which has promoted growth in the cereal bars market of 20% per year. Suitable energy intake is necessary for hormonal and metabolic function.

The consumption of carbohydrate immediately before and during exercise represents an effective strategy to provide an exogenous fuel source to the muscle and central nervous system.

As the most efficient fuel for the exercising muscles, carbohydrates are the primary source of energy during both high and low-intensity activities. The researchers believe altered zinc metabolism, coupled with increased zinc excretion and stress levels lead to fatigue and decreased endurance. Zinc has been linked to improved immune function, and as an antioxidant and anti-inflammatory, all of which can benefit hard-training athletes.

Zinc is an essential mineral that is critical to the function of many proteins and biological functions. It plays a role in growth, building and repair of muscle tissue, energy production and immune status. Diets low in animal protein, high in fibre and vegetarian diets, in particular, are associated with decreased zinc intake. Zinc status has been shown to directly affect thyroid hormone levels, BMR, and protein use, which in turn can negatively affect health and physical performance.

Dry fruits and dates have high concentrations of polyphenols with excellent nutritional value that enrich lipoprotein in plasma and protect it from oxidation. Zinc is a component of over 300 enzymes, some involved in functions important to physical performance, such as muscle energy production and protein synthesis.

Pumpkin seeds are a good source of Zinc. Nuts and seeds are widely used for their oils as well as butter and cookies. Therefore nuts and seeds are excellent nutrients for growing children and good snack for adults. A 100 gram serving of pumpkin seeds contains 7.81 milligrams of zinc. Pumpkin seeds contain big amount of zinc; a mineral very important in preventing osteoporosis. Pumpkin seeds are a very good source of Vitamin E and B vitamins. It has large amount of minerals that include copper,iron, manganese, magnesium and phosphorous. It also has antioxidant and anti-mutagenic properties and help in controlling cardiovascular diseases.

Micheletti notes that endurance athletes who adopt a diet rich in carbohydrate but low in protein and fat may decrease zinc intake, which over time may lead to a zinc deficiency with loss of body weight, latent fatigue, and decreased endurance.

The strain, an athlete puts on his/her body practicing and competing on a daily basis can lead to this deficiency, regardless of his or her age, if the zinc shortfall is not made up through diet and/or supplementation.This mineral aids in post-exertion tissue repair and in the conversion of food to fuel. Both male and female athletes have lower serum zinc levels compared with sedentary individuals. Studies correlate endurance exercise with periods of compromised immunity—zinc depletion may be one reason.

Decreases in Cardiorespiratory function, muscle strength, and endurance have been noted with poor zinc status. The Upper Limit for zinc is 40 mg. Athletes should be cautioned against single-dose zinc supplements because they often exceed this amount, and unnecessary zinc supplementation may lead to low HDL cholesterol and nutrient imbalances by interfering with absorption of other nutrients such as iron and copper.

Sports Drink

For optimal performance, athletes should aim to be hydrated and adequately fuelled during exercise. Exercise scientists have extensively researched the best fluid to drink during exercise and there is now a competitive market of beverages available that are marketed with reference to sport or performance.

Sports drinks are designed to provide the right balance of carbohydrate and fluid, to ensure that they are emptied quickly from the stomach and are rapidly absorbed from the small intestine. When used according to sports nutrition guidelines, sports drinks can have performance benefits.

Important Constituents of a Sports Drink

Carbohydrate

It is well known that consuming carbohydrate can have performance benefits in a range of sporting events. Carbohydrate provides a fuel source for muscles and the brain, and contributes to the palatability of sports drinks. Ideally the carbohydrate concentration of a sports drink should not exceed 8%, or even be slightly less. High carbohydrate solutions can impair gastric emptying during exercise.

Electrolytes

Sports drinks include the electrolytes sodium and potassium. The addition of sodium to sports drinks does have potential benefits. Sodium-containing beverages can encourage fluid intake by driving the thirst mechanism. Sodium also increases fluid absorption and retention. Sports drinks may also help with salt replacement for athletes who are heavy or salty sweaters. Most commercial sports drinks contain sodium in the range of 10-25mmol/L and in the case of some sports waters, even lower. It should be highlighted that these drinks are not suitable when rehydration is crucial to subsequent performance (i.e. must replace a fluid deficit in a short period of time).

Flavour

Flavour is an important feature of sports drinks. The more you enjoy the flavour of a drink, the more you drink. It has been shown that fluid intake via a sports drinks is significantly better when compared to plain water due to the taste.

Other Ingredients

Some beverages marketed as sports drinks have other added ingredients like vitamins, minerals, protein and herbs. The levels of antioxidants (Vitamin E and Vitamin C) in both sports drinks and sports waters in Table One provide relatively small amounts. A small number of products marketed as sports drinks contain protein. The recovery benefits of carbohydrate and protein ingestion are well documented however, the potential performance benefits of ingestion during exercise are mixed. It should be acknowledged that additional ingredients may affect the palatability, and subsequent consumption of a sports drink.

When should Sports Drinks be Used?

Before Exercise

Sports drinks may be used by athletes before an event to fine tune their fluid and fuel intake. The carbohydrate tops up muscle glycogen fuel levels, while the added sodium may reduce urine losses before exercise begins.

During Exercise

Sports drinks are primarily designed for use during exercise, for optimal fluid and fuel delivery. They will allow the athlete to perform for longer and more effectively in training and competition.

Recovery

Sports drinks assist to meet individual athletes' nutrition recovery goals by replacing fluids lost in sweat and also assist with refuelling targets to replenish glycogen stores. When aggressive re-hydration strategies are required, drinks with a higher sodium content may be more useful. To meet all recovery goals, the ingestion of sports drinks should be complimented with other foods and fluids that provide additional carbohydrate, protein, and other nutrients essential for recovery.

Fluids other than Sports Drinks

- Sports Water – A popular drink designed for those who may prefer to drink water during exercise. These drinks are lightly flavoured and generally contain a much lower carbohydrate and electrolyte content than sports drinks. May be a suitable option for moderate exercise of a short duration.
- Water – Voluntary fluid intake is less when drinking water compared to flavoured drinks. Water is suitable for low intensity or short duration (less than 45 mins) exercise, or in addition to sports drinks.
- Cordial/Soft Drink/Fruit Juice – Generally these are higher in carbohydrate and low in electrolytes compared with sports drinks. However some choices, such as cola drinks, are popular among endurance athletes as a flavor change and a small source of caffeine towards the end of a race. Such drinks should be defizzed, since carbonation decreases voluntary fluid intake and may cause gut discomfort.
- Energy Drinks – Carbohydrate concentration of these is generally too high. They contain added ingredients such as vitamins, taurine and glucuronolactone. Current evidence suggests that these additives have no impact on sport performance. However the addition of small to moderate doses of caffeine (75 - 200 mg) can help to sustain exercise performance, reduce the perception of effort, and is unlikely to alter hydration status during exercise. Caffeine is no longer banned by the World Anti Doping Agency. Ensure that you use with the advice of a sports dietitian or sports scientist and consider individual responses to caffeine.

Common Misconceptions about Sports Drinks

Sports Drinks are High in Salt

The sodium in sports drinks plays a valuable role in improving fluid absorption and the desire to drink. Sodium can also play a role in replacing the large salt losses that can occur in long events (e.g. ironman triathlons) or for salty sweaters. Sports drinks have a similar sodium content to foods such as milk, bread and breakfast cereal, but are much better tolerated during exercise.

Sports Drinks are not Suitable for Children

Children have a poor voluntary fluid intake during exercise and therefore are at greater risk of heat illness. Sports drinks have been demonstrated to improve voluntary fluid intake in children during exercise.

Sports Drinks should be Diluted

In almost all exercise situations sports drinks should not be diluted as this reduces the amount of carbohydrate available, changes the sodium concentration (both of which can affect the speed at which the drink empties from the stomach), and changes the flavour.

Sports Drinks cause Gastrointestinal Upset

You should always experiment with sports drinks in training before using them in competition. Not drinking enough sports drink, or drinking a lot in a short period of time, can cause gastrointestinal upset. Drink small amounts frequently to minimise problems.

Multivitamin

Multivitamins include a variety of vitamins and minerals, many of which are antioxidants, that help the body to run in the most efficient manner. When the body is lacking in certain nutrients, it gets weak. Bodybuilders and athletes use their body to the full, it makes sense that more than anyone, you need a good supply of vitamins. Multivitamins are actually more beneficial than you think. They affect the body for good in many different ways that are valuable to athletes and bodybuilders.

Strengthens the Immune System

Having a healthy supply of vitamins helps the body to fight off any germs or infections. Vitamin C is known for its ability to stave off the seasonal bugs but all vitamins help the body steer clear of sicknesses.

Helps with Bone and Muscle Growth

Vitamin C, vitamin K, and vitamin D, as well as magnesium and calcium, are all good for bone and joint health. The B vitamins also help to increase energy and improve your muscle recovery rate. Along with vitamin E, zinc plays an important role in helping the muscles grow.

Reduce Inflammation

Vitamin A and vitamin E both have been proven to help combat inflammation. Athletes and bodybuilders commonly have problems with inflammation of the joints or

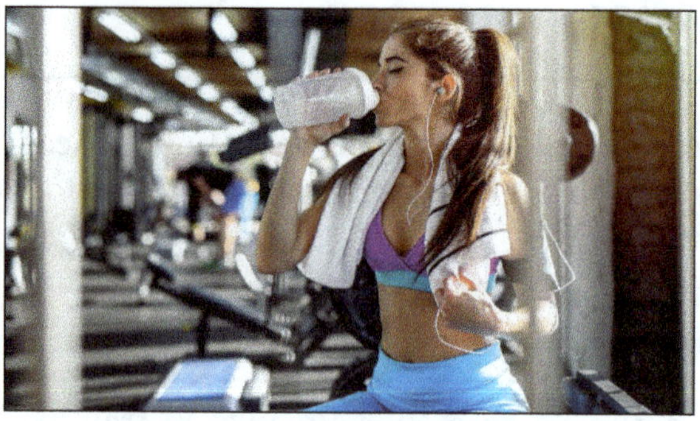

Delivers electrolytes to hydrate

Minerals such as sodium and potassium are important electrolytes needed to keep the body hydrated and replenish any lost during a sweaty training session.

Improve Memory

In-depth research was done in Australia, trying to determine if multivitamins really worked. This can be useful for athletes by helping them remember plays or game strategy and bodybuilders can remember reps and the like.

Of course, many athletes and bodybuilders have a regular day job as well, so greater memory can trickle into everyday success as well.

Less DNA Damage

Let's face it, athletes and bodybuilders love to care for their bodies, but they can also be really hard on them. It isn't easy on the body to be pushed to its limits, stretched and beat up beyond what some consider to be sane. This damage done to the body is called oxidative stress.

Multivitamins have been proven to slow the damage to the DNA, keeping you feeling younger for longer, cutting the risk of some types of cancers, and reducing the damage hard exercise can have on some organs.

This manuscript goes over how antioxidants (vitamins and minerals) help to combat the stress that exercise puts on the body.

How to take Multivitamins?

How you take your multivitamin can directly affect its effectiveness. Because many of the vitamins in a multivitamin are fat-soluble, it is always best to take your multivitamins with food. However, some vitamins, like the B vitamins are best absorbed when taken on an empty stomach.

It is also highly suggested to take your multivitamins with water. It just makes it easier to swallow and ensure it makes it all the way down the jugular.

There are several different forms of multivitamins. The most popular is the capsule or pill form. They are easy to take and don't leave any bad tastes in your mouth but some people have a hard time swallowing them.

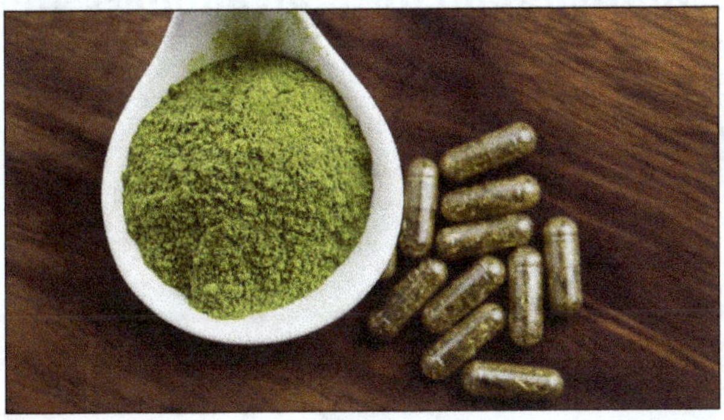

Powder forms of multivitamins are available as an alternative. At least you will know that it won't be a problem for your body to disintegrate the vitamin since it's already in powder form. Powder vitamins are also a good choice for people who have undergone gastric bypass surgery. If you do choose to use a powdered vitamin it needs to be taken stirred into water or some other drink and make sure you don't leave valuable vitamins at the bottom of the cup.

Another form of vitamins that have become popular in recent years is gummy vitamins. These are popular for kids or the kids at heart. They are more pleasant to take for sure. They are still a good option for those who have a hard time swallowing pills. Chewables are another good option as well. They actually tend to contain more vitamins than gummies because the chemical makeup of the gelatinous product sometimes rejects certain vitamins.

Lastly, you can also try liquid vitamins if none of these sound good to you. One benefit of liquid vitamins is the ability to change the dose as you please. But some vitamins actually lose their potency the longer they stay in liquid form and some need to be refrigerated, making it less convenient for travel.

What is the best Time to take Multivitamins?

Most people take their multivitamins first thing in the morning with breakfast. There are some solid reasons to take your multivitamins at this time. For one thing, it ensures that you don't forget to take it if it's done at the beginning of the day in your home. Also, it gives your body the vitamins it needs for the rest of the day, possibly aiding in setting up for an energetic and productive day.

Also, we've already touched on the fact that many vitamins are best absorbed with some healthy fats (fat-soluble vitamins like vitamins A, D, E, and K). Also, taking vitamins with a meal means the food can buffer any possible discomfort from the vitamins settling on an empty stomach.

Some vitamins will boost your energy levels, such as your B vitamins, so it wouldn't be smart to take those at night or you might have a hard time falling asleep.

How to Choose a Multivitamin for Bodybuilders and Athletes and what to Look for?

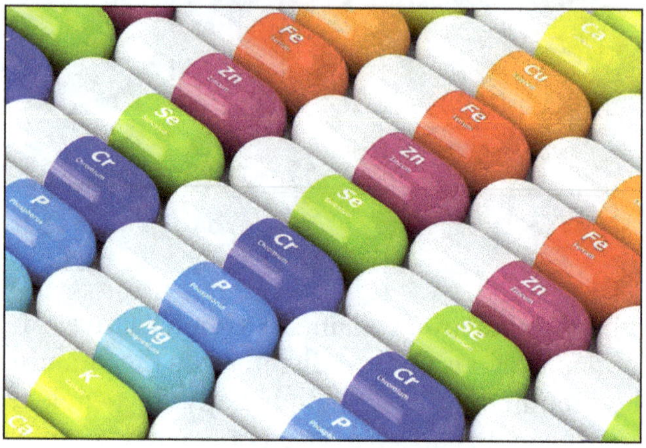

There are certain vitamins that bodybuilders and athletes should make sure to supply to their bodies. It's always best to get them through your diet but to be safe a multivitamin is a great way to ensure proper vitamin delivery. Here are the vitamins that should be included in this list:

B Complex Vitamins

There are 8 B vitamins and all of them deliver great benefits for the athlete, mostly in energy production, nerve function, and muscle tissue repair. All are water-soluble and can't be stored in the body. Vitamin B1, also known as thiamin, takes part in the conversion of glucose into energy. B2, riboflavin, also helps to produce energy but is also good for the skin.

Niacin, which is B3, converts carbs, alcohol, and fat into energy and helps to support the nervous system. Next is B5, pantothenic acid, which is mostly known to produce steroid hormones, helping with muscle growth but it also helps with metabolizing foods and alcohol.

Vitamin B6, also known as pyridoxine, also helps produce steroid hormones, metabolize carbs and protein, and help the brain processes. Biotin, B7, converts fat and glycogen into energy as well as metabolizes amino acids.

Folic acid, the vitamin form of B9, helps to distribute oxygen around the body and contributes to cell growth. Last but not least is vitamin B12. This vitamin is responsible for using amino acids and fatty acids for energy production. It also helps with nerve cell health and mental focus.

Vitamin D

Vitamin D is necessary to help absorb calcium into the body for strong bones. It also helps to build skeletal muscle and strengthen the nervous system. Also known as the sun vitamin, this vitamin is synthesized when the ultraviolet rays from the sun hit the skin. For this reason, it is especially important to take in the winter time and also by athletes living in areas where the weather is less sunny.

Vitamin D is fat-soluble and stored in the body so intake should be regulated. Excessive Vitamin D in the body can result in heart problems.

Vitamin C

This vitamin is an antioxidant, meaning that it helps to decrease the oxidative damage caused by long bouts of exercise. Oxidative stress is directly linked with an increase in free radicals, the cancer-causing cells in the body.

It is a water-soluble vitamin that cannot be produced by the body or stored. It is helpful in protein synthesis and helps build collagen levels. This is an essential part of keeping your joints and connective tissue healthy. It even helps the body to regenerate the next vitamin, Vitamin E.

Vitamin E

This is a fat-soluble vitamin that is absorbed through the liver and distributed throughout the rest of the body. This vitamin is also an antioxidant, reducing the formation of free radicals in the body, protecting it from diseases such as cancer and cardiovascular disease.

Vitamin E is also involved in strengthening the immune system and metabolism. It is also helpful to promote healthy blood flow and keeping your arteries free from blood clots.

Selenium

Yet another antioxidant to protect the body, selenium is another nutrient necessary for a healthy immune system. It is helpful for having a healthy reproduction system and thyroid gland function. An unhealthy thyroid can cause hormone imbalances and low metabolism.

Lack of selenium can cause male infertility, arthritis, and certain types of heart disease. It is also hypothesized that low selenium levels in the brain are a major cause of the cognitive decline in the elderly.

Calcium

Calcium is important for bones in three ways; for bone strength, bone repair, and bone growth. When calcium and vitamin D levels are low in the body, this can cause poor bone density that can result in fractures and weak bones. Women are more at risk of developing osteoporosis in later years. Supplementing with calcium can help to prevent this.

Calcium is also a vasodilator which means that it widens blood vessels allowing blood to flow easier and deliver oxygen and nutrients to the muscles when they need them most. This mineral also helps with nerve transmitting and hormonal secretion.

Iron

This mineral is essential for endurance exercise because it helps to form the proteins that carry oxygen throughout the body. Without this mineral, the body cannot work at maximum capacity. Your muscles will cease to contract and your lung capacity will be scant.

Endurance athletes, such as cross-country runners and cyclists, should be extra aware of their iron levels. Also, those athletes that are vegetarian or vegan should also take extra iron because most iron comes from meat or animal products and the iron that you do get from plants needs the iron you get from meat in order to be absorbed by the body.

If an iron deficiency does happen, it can take up to 6 months to reverse so it's important to check iron levels periodically and intervene as soon as possible by supplementing with iron when low levels are detected.

Zinc

This is a mineral that greatly increases the body's ability to build and repair muscle as well as produce energy. It is also helpful in strengthening the body's immune system and help fight off infection and bacteria.

As a bonus, zinc helps to regulate the senses of smell and taste.

Magnesium

This is another mineral that helps with exercise endurance. It metabolizes fat, protein, and glycolysis and helps with the cardiovascular, immune, and neuromuscular system and regulates hormonal functions.

If an athlete is low in magnesium they will notice that they can't put out effort as long as usual. This is because their body needs more oxygen to complete an intense exercise because their lack of magnesium created a deficit of blood circulation and oxygen delivery to the muscles.

Electrolytes (Sodium, Chloride, and Potassium)

Electrolytes play an important role in the body. They are called electrolytes because they are minerals that hold an electric charge.

Electrolytes are crucial when you lose water through sweating, which if you are a real athlete, you'll do a lot of that. They balance your water levels in the body and your body's pH level. This ensures that all of your organs, including the heart, the brain, and your muscles, work at optimum levels.

Bodybuilding Supplements

Creatine Monohydrate

This muscle-building, power-enhancing supplement has an extremely high safety profile and a plethora of evidence to support its efficacy. Creatine supplementation works by increasing the availability of creatine and phosphocreatine (PCr) within the muscle, helping to maintain energy during high-intensity exercise such as weightlifting. Furthermore, increasing the availability of PCr may help speed up recovery between sets.

Long-term creatine supplementation appears to enhance the quality of resistance training, generally leading to 5-15 percent greater gains in strength and performance.

Recommended dose: The fastest way to increase muscle creatine stores is to follow the loading method of 20 grams per day for 5-7 days, followed by the standard maintenance dose of 5 grams per day. However, a lower dose of 5 grams for 28 days will also increase creatine stores without causing the 2-4 pound weight gain typically seen with a loading protocol.

Caffeine

Caffeine may be the most widely used stimulant in the world, and for good reason. It has repeatedly been shown to be an effective ergogenic aid in both endurance exercise and high-intensity activity. However, when it comes to strength performance, the effects of caffeine are a little muddier.

While there's some research suggesting caffeine consumption prior to resistance training can increase one-rep max (1RM) for the bench press, other studies have found no strength benefits from caffeine.

That being said, caffeine has been shown to decrease rates of fatigue and lower perception of effort, which may be of benefit during high-intensity, high-volume workouts, or if you just need a little pick-me-up before hitting the weights.

Recommended Dose: 150-300 milligrams 30-60 minutes before your workout.

Branched Chain Amino Acids

Sipping on BCAAs between sets may help speed up the recovery and repair processes after a tough workout.

A 2010 study published in the International Journal of Sports Nutrition and Exercise Metabolism found that participants who ingested BCAAs at 100 milligrams per kilogram of bodyweight, or about 9 grams for a 200-pound individual, experienced significantly less muscle soreness and damage following a high-volume squat protocol.

It appears that BCAAs, especially leucine, help to regulate protein metabolism by promoting protein synthesis and suppressing protein degradation, which may improve recovery of muscles damaged during resistance training.

Recommended Dose: 6-10 grams before or during your workouts.

Citrulline Malate

Citrulline malate (CM) was originally marketed as an "antifatigue" supplement. In fact, if you were to travel back in time about 40 years, you'd find CM being prescribed to treat both mental and physical fatigue in post-surgery patients. More recently, CM has become popular for its performance-boosting effects.

The benefits seen with CM supplementation are most likely attributed to the synergistic combination of both L-citrulline and malate, which may help to increase rates of ATP during exercise, followed by increased rates of PCr recovery after exercise.

Previous investigations have shown that a single dose of CM (8 grams) increased the number of repetitions performed during an upper-body resistance training protocol and reduced soreness at 24 and 48 hours post-exercise (compared to a placebo).7 Recently, researchers from Mississippi State University found that a single dose of CM (8 grams) significantly increased the number of lower-body repetitions compared to a placebo group.

CM may be beneficial in improving exercise performance during upper- and lower-body multiple-bout resistance exercise in resistance-trained men.

Recommended Dose: 8 grams of CM taken 60 minutes before exercise.

No Boosters

Nitrate-rich foods like beets, radishes, and pomegranates are a great way to boost the production of nitric oxide (NO). Although there's very limited research examining the effects of beet root juice and pomegranate extract on resistance training, these ingredients have previously been shown to increase skeletal muscle blood flow and lead to reduced soreness, which may ultimately lead to improvements in strength and performance.

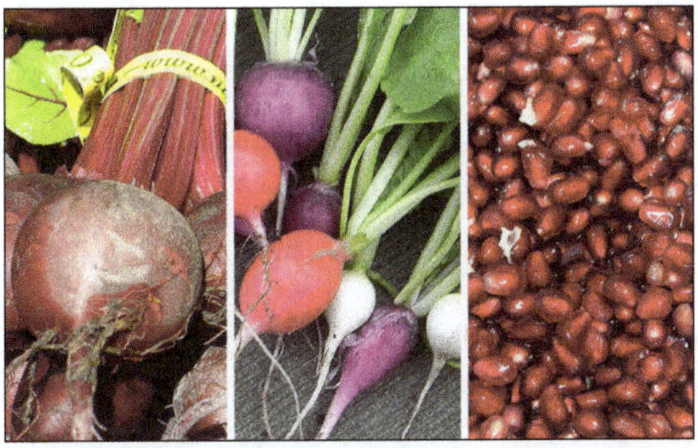

Nitrate-rich foods like beets, radishes, and pomegranates are a great way to boost the production of nitric oxide (NO).

Several studies have used either beet root juice or pomegranate extract in multi-ingredient performance supplements and have observed improvements in strength, hypertrophy, and performance in resistance-trained men. At this point, however, it's difficult to determine if these benefits are from beet root juice and pomegranate extract working alone or synergistically with other ingredients.

Recommended Dose: 500 milligrams of beet root juice or pomegranate extract 30-60 minutes before your workout.

Whey Protein

Fast-digesting protein like whey is optimal post-workout as it can help improve your muscles' ability to recover and adapt after strenuous exercise. In fact, consumption of whey protein has been found to stimulate muscle protein synthesis to a greater degree than other proteins like casein and soy.

The benefits of protein supplementation and showed that supplementing with protein during prolonged (greater than 6 weeks) resistance-type training can lead to significantly greater increases in muscle mass and strength when compared to resistance training without a dietary protein intervention.

Blends of protein, like whey and casein, have been shown to promote muscle hypertrophy and improve body composition to a greater extent than soy-based proteins when consumed after resistance exercise.

The combination of fast-digesting whey and slow-digesting casein keep the body in a highly anabolic environment for a prolonged period of time, helping to keep rates of protein synthesis up, while minimizing any muscle breakdown.

Lifters who follow high-volume or high-intensity resistance-training programs, as many bodybuilders do, may also benefit from carbohydrate intake immediately post-workout. Compared with a placebo, carbohydrates combined with protein immediately postworkout and one hour after a bout of resistance exercise have been shown to increase insulin levels and rates of glycogen resynthesis.

Recommended Dose: 20-30 grams of whey (or whey/casein blend) protein with a high-glycemic carbohydrate post-workout.

Glutamine

While this nonessential amino acid may not deliver earth-shattering PRs or extreme muscle growth, it does play an important role in repair and recovery. Glutamine works by removing excess ammonia, which can accumulate during intense exercise, helping to regulate your body's acid-base balance. Individuals who are engaged in heavy resistance training, two-a-day training splits, or are in a calorie deficit may benefit from the extra support of glutamine supplementation.

Recommended Dose: 20-30 grams a day, consuming 10 grams post-workout.

Fish Oils

Fish oils are an excellent source of omega-3 fatty acids, which provide myriad benefits for the body. For strength athletes and bodybuilders, we're most concerned with their anti-inflammatory and antioxidant properties. Intense resistance training can cause microscopic tears in your muscle fibers, leading to muscle damage and inflammation. While some inflammation is desirable, too much can delay the post-exercise recovery process.

Research suggests that omega-3 fatty acids can help reduce post-exercise muscle soreness and speed up the recovery process, getting you ready for your next session with the weights. As an added benefit, when combined with BCAAs and carbs, omega-3s can increase protein synthesis rates, leading to greater gains in muscle mass.

Recommended Dose: 2 grams daily, ideally with a meal.

References

- 150-dietary-assessment-methods-for-the-athlete-pros-and-cons-of-different-methods, sports-science-exchange: gssiweb.org, Retrieved 14 March, 2019
- Sports-Drinks: sportsdietitians.com.au, Retrieved 23 May, 2019
- Best-multivitamins-bodybuilders-athletes: workoutuni.com,
- The-8-supplements-for-strength-athletes-and-bodybuilders: bodybuilding.com, Retrieved 18 January, 2019
- AnanthanPadmashree, K.S. Gopal, A.S. Kadaba, S.B. Amarinder, Development of shelf stable protein rich composite cereal bar. Journal of Food Science and Technology, 49, 2012, 335-341

5

Sports Psychology

An interdisciplinary science that integrates the concepts of physiology, kinesiology, biomechanics and psychology is referred to as sports psychology. Performance anxiety, aggression in sport, psychological susceptibility to injury, body image and self-esteem are sub-fields of this science. This chapter discusses in detail these theories related to sports psychology.

Psychology of Sport

The specialized field of sports psychology has developed rapidly in recent years. The importance of a sports psychologist as an integral member of the coaching and health care teams is widely recognized. Sports psychologists can teach skills to help athletes enhance their learning process and motor skills, cope with competitive pressures, fine-tune the level of awareness needed for optimal performance, and stay focused amid the many distractions of team travel and in the competitive environment. Psychological training should be an integral part of an athlete's holistic training process, carried out in conjunction with other training elements. This is best accomplished by a collaborative effort among the coach, the sport psychologist, and the athlete; however, a knowledgeable and interested coach can learn basic psychological skills and impart them to the athlete, especially during actual practice.to help the parties' air and resolve differences.

Preparing for Competition

Simple psychological skills to help the athlete manage the competitive performance environment include:

- Learning relaxation skills (e.g. Progressive relaxation, slow, controlled, deep abdominal breathing or autogenic training.
- Mastering all of the attentional styles (types of concentration).
- Imagery (both visualization and kinesthetic).
- Self talk.
- Developing a precomputations mental routine to be employed immediately prior to competition on game day.

Injured Athlete

Injured athletes commonly experience at least three emotional responses: isolation, frustration and disturbances of mood. The Sports Psychologist in consultation with the medical team must make ready the injured athlete to participate in sports and games.

The following points the importance of sports psychology:

Enhancement of Physiological Capacities

Sports psychology plays a very unique role in the enhancement of physiological capacities such as strength, speed and flexibility etc., Motivation plays a major role in the enhancement of physical capacity of sport persons. It is well-known as well as an established fact that psychological capacities or powers can increase physiological capacities of individuals.

Learning the Motor Skills

Sports psychology plays its major role in the learning of motor skills. Motor skills learning depends on the individual's level of readiness, i.e., physiological readiness and psychological readiness. Physiological readiness in children is development of the necessary strength, flexibility and endurance as well as the development of various organ systems so that they may perform motor skills required in the activity. Psychological readiness is related to the learner's state of mind. It means the desire and willingness to learn the particular skill. In psychological readiness, sports psychology plays an important role. Sports psychology is also helpful in the cognitive stage, the social-active stage and the autonomous stage of motor skill learning.

Understanding the Behavior

Sports psychology helps in understanding the behavior of athletes or sportspersons engaged in competitive sports. Coaches also come to know the interest, attitude towards physical activity, instincts, drives and personality of sportspersons. It does not play its role only in understanding of behavior but it also plays its role in medication of behavior in various sports situations.

Controlling the Emotions

Sports psychology plays a very important role in controlling the emotions of sportspersons during practice as well as competition. Generally, these emotions may bring spontaneous changes in the behavior of sportspersons. These are anger, disgust, gear, negative self-thinking and feeling of ownership, etc. If these emotions are not controlled well in time, the performance may be decreased. Sports psychology plays a vital role at such juncture. It helps in balancing the arousal of emotions which further improves the performance.

Preparation of Athletes Psychologically for Competitions

Sports psychology also plays its role in preparation of athletes psychologically for competitions. Intact, it has become a trend to give psychological tips to athletes or team players before and after the competitions. That is why, sports psychologists' services are required with a national level and international level terms. They create the will 'to win' in the players.

Role in the Emotional Problems of Sports Persons

Stress, tension and anxiety are natural during practice period and competitions or tournaments. There may be some other emotional problems such as depression, frustration. Anorexia and panic etc. The knowledge of sports psychology may be helpful in such situations. Techniques of relaxation and concentration for stress management can be applied on sportspersons who are under such problems. Conclusively, it can be said that sports psychology plays a very vital role in enhancing the performance of sportspersons. It deals with the various mental qualities such as concentration, confidence, emotional control and commitment etc., which are important for successful performance in sports and games.

Motivational Techniques for Coaches and Athletes

Goal Setting

Goal setting is the process of systematically planning ways to achieve specific accomplishments within a certain amount of time. Research suggests that goals should be specific, measurable, difficult but attainable, time-based, written down, and a combination of short-term and long-term goals. A meta-analysis of goal setting in sport suggests that when compared to setting no goals or "do your best" goals, setting the above types of goals is an effective method for improving performance. According to Dr. Eva V. Monsma, short-term goals should be used to help achieve long-term goals. Dr. Monsma also states that it is important to "set goals in positive terms by focusing on behaviors that should be present rather than those that should be absent." Each long-term goal should also have a series of short-term goals that progress in difficulty. For instance, short-term goals should progress from those that are easy to achieve to those that are more challenging. Having challenging short-term goals will remove the repetitiveness of easy goals and will give one an edge when striving for their long-term goals.

Imagery

Imagery (or motor imagery) can be defined as using multiple senses to create or recreate experiences in one's mind.

Additionally, the more vivid images are, the more likely they are to be interpreted by the brain as identical to the actual event, which increases the effectiveness of mental practice with imagery. Good imagery, therefore, attempts to create as lifelike an image as possible through the use of multiple senses (e.g., sight, smell), proper timing, perspective, and accurate portrayal of the task. Both anecdotal evidence from athletes and research findings suggest imagery is an effective tool to enhance performance and psychological states relevant to performance (e.g., confidence). This is a concept commonly used by coaches and athletes the day before an event.

Pre-performance Routines

Pre-performance routines refer to the actions and behaviors athletes use to prepare for a game or performance. This includes pregame routines, warm up routines, and actions an athlete will regularly do, mentally and physically, before they execute the performance. Frequently, these will incorporate other commonly used techniques, such as imagery or self-talk. Examples would be visualizations done by skiers, dribbling by basketball players at the foul line, and pre shot routines golfers or baseball players use prior to a shot or pitch. These routines help to develop consistency and predictability for the player. This allows the muscles and mind to develop better motor control.

Self-talk

Self-talk refers to the thoughts and words athletes and performers say to themselves, usually in their minds. Self-talk phrases are used to direct attention towards a particular thing in order to improve focus or are used alongside other techniques to facilitate their effectiveness. For example, a softball player may think "release point" when at bat to direct her attention to the point where the pitcher releases the ball, while a golfer may say "smooth stroke" before putting to stay relaxed. Research suggests either positive or negative self-talk may improve performance, suggesting the effectiveness of self-talk phrases depends on how the phrase is interpreted by the individual. However, the use of positive self-talk is considered to be more efficacious and is consistent with the associative network theory of Gordon Bower and the self-efficacy tenet within the broader Social Cognitive Theory of Albert Bandura. The use of words in sport has been widely utilized. The ability to bombard the unconscious mind with one single positive phrase, is one of the most effective and easy to use psychological skills available to any athlete.

Using Extrinsic Rewards

The key aspect in using extrinsic rewards effectively is that they reinforce an athlete's sense of competence and self-worth. Thus, a reward should be informational in nature rather than controlling. If a reward comes to be controlling, it can significantly undermine intrinsic motivation. For a reward to be informational, it is advisable that it has relatively little monetary worth (i.e. it is a token reward), such as a 'woman of the match' or 'athlete of the tour' title. Also, the reward should be presented to an athlete in front of all potential recipients with some emphasis placed on the prestige associated with it. Other popular ways of using token rewards include etching athletes' names on annual honors boards for their contributions, or awarding a special item of clothing.

Motivational Music

A particularly good way to motivate athletes in training and prior to competition is through the use of music they perceive to be inspirational.

Importance of Sports Psychology

1. Sport psychology helps you understand yourself as an athlete:

You need to have mental strategies for learning, practice and performance factors. Sport psychology gives you the methods and approaches to become aware of what you need so you and your coach can craft custom interventions.

2. Sport psychology helps you work better with your parents:

Your parents should be part of your success team, at least at some level. It does not necessarily mean they should coach you, but it would be nice to have a solid relationship with them, and excellent communication skills so they can assist you in your career.

3. Sport psychology helps you work better with your coaches:

Your coach is perhaps the most important person on your team. You need a great working relationship with this person. Sport psychology can help you create this relationship, and nurture it.

4. Sport psychology helps you navigate your sport career:

There are many blind alleys, pitfalls and false paths in a sport career. Sport psychology helps you create a vision for success, and goals and objectives, so you can execute that master plan.

5. Sport psychology helps you prepare your mind:

It is critical that you know how to prepare mentally and emotionally for lessons, practices and performances. Sport psychology helps you devise a customized mental readiness process that helps you transition from your normal work, school or social worlds into the special world of competition.

6. Sport psychology helps you concentrate so you can enter the zone:

Attentional control is psychologist-speak for concentration or focus. Sport psychology helps you create strong control over where and how you place your attention so you can concentrate on the proper attentional cues, and you are able to block out unwanted, distracting cues.

7. Sport psychology helps you bounce back from setbacks:

It is critical that you become resilient to the inevitable problems and set-backs that competitive sport brings. You need solid mental toughness that helps you refocus, reset and re-energize for what is to come.

8. Sport psychology helps you increase motivation and drive:

Successful athletes who have long careers fuel them with exciting goals, a vision for the legacy they want to leave, and dreams of how they want to play. Sport psychology helps you craft engaging goals that create positive energy within you, so you have huge amounts of drive and determination to achieve your potential.

9. Sport psychology helps you handle stress and pressure:

One of the major ways sport psychology helps you is through stress reduction in learning and performance. While some stress is inevitable and natural, levels of stress that are excessive damage performance. Sport psychology helps you manage stress and turn it into success.

10. Sport psychology helps you handle the paradox of success:

An issue that every athlete faces at some time is the paradox of success. As you become more successful, there are more pressures and more distractions pulling at you. Sport psychology helps you address these, stay focused, and helps you continue to sustain your best performances.

Performance Anxiety

Performance anxiety symptoms are often present in athletes. While some people become "pumped up" during the competition, if you interpret the rush of adrenaline as anxiety and negative thoughts take over, this can interfere with your ability to perform.

Performance Anxiety and Sports Psychology

People with social anxiety disorder (SAD) fear social and performance situations. The most common fear is public speaking. However, other types of performances such as musical and athletic may also lead to anxiety.

Sport psychology is a division of psychology aimed at better preparing the mind of an athlete for competition. Most sport psychologists work with athletes to help them overcome anxiety about performance during competitions. In its most extreme form, this type of anxiety would be diagnosed as SAD.

Performance Anxiety and Athletic Performance

Anxiety before or during athletic competitions can interfere with your performance as an athlete. The coordinated movement required by athletic events becomes increasingly difficult when your body is in a tense state. While a certain level of physical arousal is helpful and prepares us for competition, when the physical symptoms of anxiety are too great, they may seriously interfere with your ability to compete.

A certain amount of worry about how you perform can be helpful in competition. At the same time, negative thought patterns and expectations of failure can bring about a self-fulfilling prophecy.

If there is a large difference between how you fare during practice and how you do during competitions, anxiety may be affecting your performance.

Sports Performance Anxiety Triggers

Some types of athletes are more prone to feeling the effects of anxiety on performance. As an amateur athlete, you are more likely than seasoned professionals to experience anxiety that interferes with your ability to perform in competition. This makes sense due to your relative lack of experience both in competition and in managing feelings of being "pumped up".

If you are an athlete who participates in individual sports, you are also more likely to experience anxiety than those who play team sports. It makes sense that being part of a team helps to manage some of the pressure that you feel when you compete alone.

Finally, there is evidence that in team sports, if your team plays at the venue of the opposition (known as an "away" game), anxiety levels tend to be higher than when your team is playing at home. Again, it makes sense that having greater fan support and being more familiar with the location helps to reduce anxiety.

Athletes who Thrive under Pressure

Research shows that self-confidence plays a role in how you respond to symptoms of anxiety during athletic performance. If you are confident in your ability, you are more likely to have a positive reaction to being "pumped up" and will thrive on the challenge of competition. Elite athletes are often so focused on their behavior that they interpret arousal as excitement rather than anxiety.

In general, self-confidence tends to be highest when you believe in your ability and feel that you have properly prepared for a competition.

Worry and confidence are at opposite ends of the spectrum; when confidence is strong, it tends to crowd worry out of the mind.

Managing Performance Anxiety Symptoms

There are a number of strategies you can employ to reduce performance anxiety symptoms, such as the following:

- Reduce negative thought patterns that contribute to anxiety through cognitive restructuring (self-help books on cognitive-behavioral therapy will help with this).
- Learn how to interpret arousal during the competition as positive or acceptable rather than negative (self-help books on acceptance and commitment therapy will help with this).
- Ensure that you have practiced enough so that you are confident during competition.
- Generate that "team spirit" even for individual sports by making friends with other competitors.
- For "away" games, ask friends or family to be there to root you on.

Aggression in Sport

Aggression has a long history in both sport and nonsport contexts. There is some variation in the definitions of aggression employed by different people. However, it is commonly agreed that aggression is a verbal or physical behavior that is directed intentionally toward another individual and has the potential to cause psychological or physical harm. In addition, the target of the behavior should be motivated to avoid such treatment. Typically, definitions of aggression incorporate the notion of intent to cause harm; that is, for behavior to be classified as aggressive, the perpetrator must have the intent to harm the victim. However, strict behavioral definitions of aggression exclude the term intent because it refers to an internal state, which cannot be observed.

Aggression has been distinguished between instrumental and hostile. Instrumental aggression is a behavior directed at the target as a means to an end, for example, injuring a player to gain a competitive advantage, or late tackling to stop an opponent from scoring. Thus, instrumental aggression is motivated by some other goal. In contrast, hostile aggression is a behavior aimed toward another person who has angered or provoked the individual and is an end in itself. Its purpose is to harm for its own sake, for example, hitting an opponent who has just been aggressive against the player. Hostile aggression is typically preceded by anger. Instrumental aggression, in pursuit of a goal, is not normally associated with anger and, in sport, is far more frequent than hostile aggression. In both types of aggression, a target person is harmed, and the harm can be physical or psychological.

Aggression, Assertion and Intent

In sport, the word aggressive is often used when assertive is more appropriate. For example, coaches describe strong physical play as aggressive, when this type of play is actually assertive; it is within the rules of the game and there is no intention to cause harm. The difference between aggression and assertion lies in the intention to harm. If there is no intent to harm the opponent, and the athlete is using legitimate means to achieve goals, the behavior is assertive, not aggressive. When one is being assertive, the intention is to establish dominance rather than to harm the opponent. Behaviors such as tackling in rugby, checking in ice hockey, and breaking up a double play in baseball may be seen as assertive as long as these are performed as legal components of the contest and without malice. However, these same actions would represent aggression if the athlete's intention was to cause injury.

It is often difficult to distinguish aggression from assertion in sport. Although assertive behaviors are forceful behaviors that are not intended to injure the victim, by their nature, they may result in unintended harm to the athlete's opponent. In addition, some sports involve forceful physical contact, which has the capacity to harm another person, but this contact is within the rules of sport. Assertive behaviors have also been labeled sanctioned aggression. Thus, sanctioned aggression is any behavior that falls within a particular sport's rules or is widely accepted as such: for example, using the shoulder to force a player off the ball in soccer and tackling below the shoulders in rugby. Examples are combat sports, such as judo, karate, and wrestling, and team contact sports, such as rugby, ice hockey, American football, and lacrosse. Perhaps the confusion between assertion and aggression arises because both have the capacity to harm the target, although, as noted earlier, only aggression involves intention to harm.

Incorporating the notion of intent in definitions of aggression has the difficulty of establishing which behavior is aggressive. This is because the only person knowing whether there is intent to cause harm is the person who carries out the action. Two features of definitions of aggression that have not been questioned are the capacity of behavior to cause harm and the intentional (nonaccidental) nature of the behavior.

Psychological Susceptibility to Injury

Sport and recreational-related injuries have become a significant public health concern for physically active persons. For example, in 2006 the Centers for Disease Control and Prevention estimated that participation in high school sports will result in approximately 1.4 million injuries reported to medical staff at a rate of 2.4 injuries per 1,000 athlete exposures (i.e., practices or competitions). As sport and other physical activities continue to be promoted as part of maintaining and restoring health, there will continue to be an increase in sport-related injuries. These trends have resulted in multifactorial perspectives of injury prediction and prevention. Advances in safety of equipment, improvement to the physical environment, and new policies to protect sport participants have been implemented. Of relevance to this resource, but not likely as well known, are those approaches that involve the monitoring and modifying of psychological factors associated with sport injury.

Psychological Stress and Sports-related Injury

In the 1960s, Thomas Holmes and colleagues suggested that changes in social stress, as measured by assessing accumulated stressful life events, were a precursor to changes in overall health. Essentially, life events often evoked changes in psychological status that required increased efforts to cope. This response to stress, or stress reactivity, was the mechanism underpinning the relationship between stress and health, whereby as stress demands and coping efforts increased, health would be compromised (e.g., onset of illness, progression of disease). In the1970s, Holmes and later S. T. Bramwell and colleagues were the first to explore this notion in sport. They surveyed American football players and found greater levels of stress were associated with increased likelihood of athletic injury. This prompted further exploration of the relationship between stress and sport injury, yet much of what followed failed to replicate Holmes and Bramwell's findings.

Model of Stress and Injury

The stress-injury model posits that three categories of psychological risk factors (i.e., personality, history of stress, and coping resources) influence athletes' response to stressful athletic situations that, in turn, influences the likelihood of athletic injury through various stress-response mechanisms. In addition to proposing psychological risk factors, their model offered specific avenues for psychological interventions and skills training to buffer adverse stress-related consequences for athletes' health and to minimize, or ideally prevent, athletic injury.

Stress Response Mechanisms

Cognitive Appraisal

Central to the stress and injury model is one's cognitive appraisal. Based upon the pioneering work of Richard Lazarus and Susan Folkman, the cognitive appraisal involves a balance (or imbalance) between two perceptions. The primary appraisal reflects perceived demands or threat of the stressor whereas the secondary appraisal reflects perceived personal and situational resources to cope with those demands and threat. When coping resources are perceived to be adequate to manage threat or demands, stress reactivity is minimal. In contrast, an imbalance occurs where one's perception of stress demands exceeds available coping resources, at which point stress reactivity is heightened.

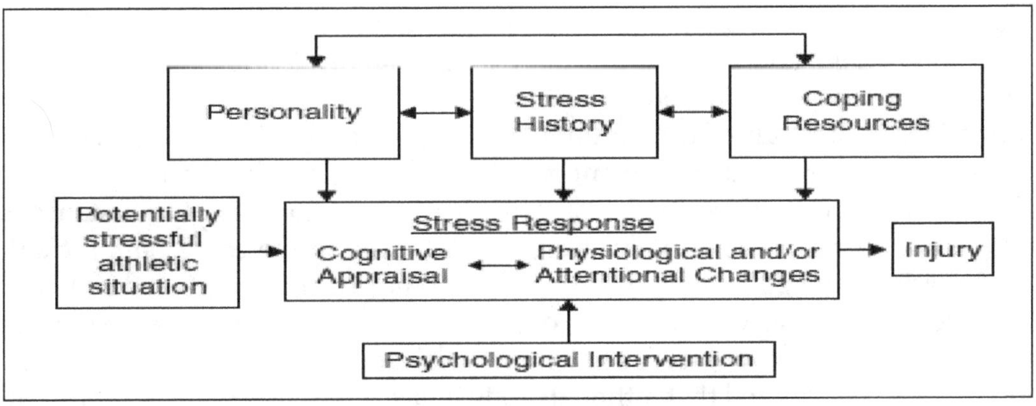

Stress and injury model.

Physiological Considerations

Very little attention has been given to physiological considerations. Within the model, stress responses that were initially described involved increase in muscle tension, which was thought to potentially impair motor control and slow reaction time (RT) that, in turn, may heighten injury vulnerability when engaged in sport competition and/or training. Over time, three additional pathways emerged associating psychological stress to physiological response. Perturbations in visual attention involving peripheral narrowing of visual field were described among highly stressed athletes and were hypothesized to heighten risk for injury (i.e., being blindsided). The other pathways linking stress to injury involved excess autonomic activity (e.g., increases in stress hormones) that were posited to increase injury risk by impairing immune function and other cellular processes necessary for muscle repair following strenuous exercise training, or by altering sleep and associated secretion of growth factors also required for muscle anabolism. To date, excess elevation in psychological stress-related autonomic activity remains as the leading mechanism associated with athletic injury, but the specific causal pathway(s) remains unknown.

Body Image and Self-esteem

Body image and self-esteem, considered synonymous with self-worth, is a global and relatively stable construct that reflects a person's evaluation about self-concept, that is, the set of beliefs and cognitions about one's qualities, character, roles, and attributes. Body image and self-esteem is a complex and multifaceted concept of the self, and arguably one of the most important facets of body image and self-esteem in Westernized countries is a sense of self that is focused on the body or physique. Specifically, body image and self-esteem is a strong predictor of global body image and self-esteem when individuals value how they look and feel physically—meaning how one feels about one's physique, form, and function is a predominant guide to how one feels about oneself more globally. Body image and self-esteem, also identified as physical self-worth or physical body image and self-esteem, is defined as an evaluation about the appearance and functioning of one's body. Theorists consider that body image and self-esteem develops as a result of the evaluative perceptions that arise from the different domains, such as perceived sport competence, physical condition, attractiveness, and weight concern. In turn, these arise from the different subdomains. For instance, positive self-evaluations of upper body strength contribute to the corresponding subdomain of physical strength, which in turn would enhance body image and self-esteem. On the other hand, negative evaluations of soccer competence will decrease the related subdomain of sport competence, and then in physical body image and self-esteem. In addition, it has been argued that although body image and self-esteem may be relatively stable over time, specific self-evaluations may fluctuate depending on the situational cues—an individual may feel better about personal physical stamina after completing a 10-mile run or worse if unable to complete this run.

Researchers suggest that it is during adolescence that body image and self-esteem becomes particularly salient as a result of the physical and social changes associated with this developmental stage. Furthermore, researchers have also shown that there are gender differences in body image and self-esteem during this period and across adulthood, whereby men have reported higher levels of body image and self-esteem than women. While there are various potential reasons for this, many researchers have proposed that the greater sociocultural pressures on women to be thin, their inability to attain this standard, and the negative stereotyping of those whose current body is discrepant from the idealized standard, may partly explain this difference. Nonetheless, high body image and self-esteem is desirable in both sexes because it has a powerful influence on men and women's psychological, physical, and social well-being. Essentially, individuals who have higher levels of body image and self-esteem are more likely to report higher well-being in these domains. As a result, researchers have highlighted the importance of exploring factors that may increase or maintain body image and self-esteem because it has public health importance. One such factor is exercise.

Body Image and Self-esteem and Exercise Research

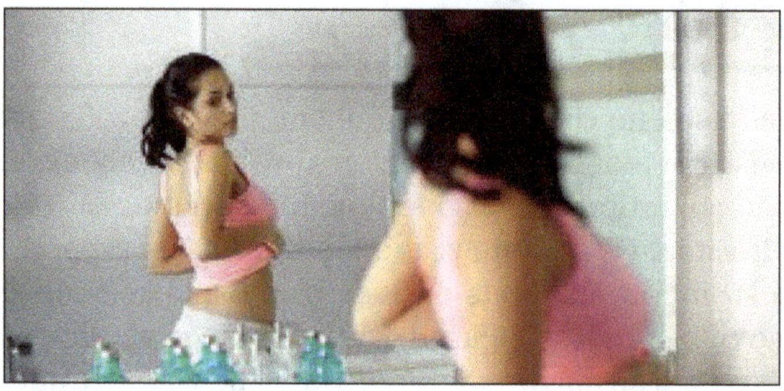

Given that exercise has been consistently associated with psychological benefits, there has been an enduring interest in establishing the potential benefits of exercise as a strategy for the enhancement of body image and self-esteem, and more specifically body image and self-esteem. With the use of different measures like specific cognitive and affective questions (Body Esteem Scale) and figure ratings (silhouettes that gradually increase in size and shape), researchers have found that exercise and body image and self-esteem are reciprocally related across the lifespan and in many diverse populations. This means that individuals suffering from low body image and self-esteem will be less likely to be physically active, and that individuals being more physically active show higher body image and self-esteem levels.

Often in research studies focused on body image and self-esteem improvements, the exercise parameters assessed have differed markedly. Specifically, the duration and intensity of training sessions, the number of training sessions per week, or the length of the training program tested varied from one study to another. It is possible that body image and self-esteem improvements found following exercise might be restricted to one particular type (aerobic training, strength training) or intensity (light, moderate, vigorous). However, at this point, it is not possible to provide an indication for the specific doses or types of exercise necessary to enhance body image and self-esteem. Thus, these parameters of exercise seem to be an important consideration for future research.

Another important problem is that some researchers are still using measures of global body image and self-esteem such as the Rosenberg body image and self-esteem scale. This approach implicitly assumes that the overall concept of body image and self-esteem would be related to exercise, which may not be the case, and lead to the erroneous conclusions that exercise is ineffective in improving body image and self-esteem. Therefore, it is important to move beyond global measures and adopt a more systematic assessment of body image and self-esteem since exercise might have a more meaningful influence on this aspect of body image and self-esteem without affecting others related to global body image and self-esteem.

References

- How-do-i-handle-performance-anxiety-as-an-athlete-3024337: verywellmind.com, Retrieved 15 April, 2019
- Aggression-in-sport, sports-psychology: psychology.iresearchnet.com, Retrieved 17 March, 2019
- Psychological-susceptibility-to-injury, sports-psychology: psychology.iresearchnet.com, Retrieved 14 February, 2019
- Body-image-and-self-esteem, sports-psychology: psychology.iresearchnet.com, Retrieved 25 June, 2019
- Vealey RS. P3 thinking. In Vealey, RS. Ed., Coaching for the Inner Edge. Morgantown, WV: Fitness Information Technology, 2005, 201-224.

Permissions

All chapters in this book are published with permission under the Creative Commons Attribution Share Alike License or equivalent. Every chapter published in this book has been scrutinized by our experts. Their significance has been extensively debated. The topics covered herein carry significant information for a comprehensive understanding. They may even be implemented as practical applications or may be referred to as a beginning point for further studies.

We would like to thank the editorial team for lending their expertise to make the book truly unique. They have played a crucial role in the development of this book. Without their invaluable contributions this book wouldn't have been possible. They have made vital efforts to compile up to date information on the varied aspects of this subject to make this book a valuable addition to the collection of many professionals and students.

This book was conceptualized with the vision of imparting up-to-date and integrated information in this field. To ensure the same, a matchless editorial board was set up. Every individual on the board went through rigorous rounds of assessment to prove their worth. After which they invested a large part of their time researching and compiling the most relevant data for our readers.

The editorial board has been involved in producing this book since its inception. They have spent rigorous hours researching and exploring the diverse topics which have resulted in the successful publishing of this book. They have passed on their knowledge of decades through this book. To expedite this challenging task, the publisher supported the team at every step. A small team of assistant editors was also appointed to further simplify the editing procedure and attain best results for the readers.

Apart from the editorial board, the designing team has also invested a significant amount of their time in understanding the subject and creating the most relevant covers. They scrutinized every image to scout for the most suitable representation of the subject and create an appropriate cover for the book.

The publishing team has been an ardent support to the editorial, designing and production team. Their endless efforts to recruit the best for this project, has resulted in the accomplishment of this book. They are a veteran in the field of academics and their pool of knowledge is as vast as their experience in printing. Their expertise and guidance has proved useful at every step. Their uncompromising quality standards have made this book an exceptional effort. Their encouragement from time to time has been an inspiration for everyone.

The publisher and the editorial board hope that this book will prove to be a valuable piece of knowledge for students, practitioners and scholars across the globe.

Index

www.ingramcontent.com/pod-product-compliance
Lightning Source LLC
LaVergne TN
LVHW080603210926
848485LV00003B/98